Family Support and Family Caregiving across Disabilities

Family members provide the majority of care for individuals with disabilities in the United States. Recognition is growing that family caregiving deserves and requires societal support, and evidence-based practices have been established for reducing stress associated with caregiving. Despite the substantial research literature on family support that has developed, researchers, advocates and professionals have often worked in separate categorical domains such as family support for caregiving for the frail elderly, for individuals with mental illness, or for people with development disabilities.

Family Support and Family Caregiving across Disabilities addresses this significant limitation through cross-categorical and lifespan analyses of family support and family caregiving from the perspectives of theory and conceptual frameworks, empirical research, and frameworks and recommendations for improvements in public policy. The book also examines children with disabilities, children with autism, adults with schizophrenia, and individuals with cancer across the life cycle.

This book was published as a two-part special issue in the *Journal of Family Social Work*.

George H. S. Singer is based at the University of California, Santa Barbara, USA.

David E. Biegel is based at Case Western Reserve University, USA.

Patricia Conway is based at Essentia Institute of Rural Health, Duluth, MN, USA.

Family Support and Family Caregiving across Disabilities

Edited by
George H. S. Singer, David E. Biegel and Patricia Conway

Routledge
Taylor & Francis Group
LONDON AND NEW YORK

First published 2012
by Routledge
2 Park Square, Milton Park, Abingdon, Oxfordshire OX14 4RN

Simultaneously published in the USA and Canada
by Routledge
711 Third Avenue, New York, NY 10017

First issued in paperback 2014

Routledge is an imprint of the Taylor & Francis Group, an informa business

This book is a reproduction of the *Journal of Family Social Work*, vol. 12, issue 2 and vol. 13, issue 3. The Publisher requests to those authors who may be citing this book to state, also, the bibliographical details of the special issue on which the book was based.

British Library Cataloguing in Publication Data
A catalogue record for this book is available from the British Library

ISBN13: 978-0-415-68268-8 (hbk)
ISBN13: 978-1-138-00898-4 (pbk)

Typeset in Times New Roman
by Taylor & Francis Books

Disclaimer
The publisher would like to make readers aware that the chapters in this book are referred to as articles as they had been in the special issue. The publisher accepts responsibility for any inconsistencies that may have arisen in the course of preparing this volume for print.

Contents

Part III: Public Policy

Introduction: An Overview of Family Support and Family Caregiving across Disabilities

DAVID E. BIEGEL
Mandel School of Applied Social Sciences, Case Western University, Cleveland, Ohio

GEORGE H. S. SINGER
Gevirtz Graduate School of Education, University of California, Santa Barbara, California

PATRICIA CONWAY
Essentia Institute of Rural Health, Duluth, MN

Over the past two decades, attention has increased regarding the role that families play in providing support to their family members with physical, cognitive, or psychiatric impairments and disabilities. This attention has resulted in a rich and growing literature on family caregiving and family support as reflected by the chapters in this book. The book's nine chapters are organized into three sections—Conceptual Frameworks, Empirical Research, and Public Policy. In this overview, we present major themes and issues in each of these three areas and brief summaries of the content of the book's chapters.

Part I: Conceptual Frameworks

The first section of this book focuses on major premises in research on family caregiving and family support. A re-evaluation of theories of family caregiving is timely for several reasons. Major societal changes in the past half century raise the question of whether or not research paradigms launched in the 1970's need to be reviewed to determine if they are malleable and durable in a changed environment. Early theories and studies appeared in number initially in the mid 1970's. During this era a dominant paradigm was established, the stress and coping perspective. It defined having family members with disabilities as stressors and caregiving as burdensome, resulting in physical and psychological distress. The stress, coping, and crisis framework has guided hundreds of caregiving studies and generated a considerable knowledge base. However, the past four decades have been marked by transformation in the make-up of families, societal assumptions about who should provide care, views of help giving, and the aims of family support.

Feminism, multiculturalism, and the positive psychology movement have altered the intellectual context. As a result, ideas that have previously been taken for granted have been challenged, including the assumption that mothers and daughters should perform almost all of the unpaid caregiving for their relatives. Many women no longer accept that caregiving is an inevitable part of their gender role. Men are increasingly active as caregivers but they are far from providing an equal share of caregiving. Another important shift has been the undermining of the once pervasive belief that caregiving has only negative impacts on family care providers. A more contemporary view is that there is a wide range in variability in the ways caregiving for a relative with a disability impacts caregivers. This expanded range includes positive views of the caregiving experience. The general emphasis on pathology in the social sciences has been eroded by the positive psychology movement. Researchers have begun studying successful families and trying to account for the conditions which promote resilience, well-being and perceptions of benefit for both caregivers and care recipients. This change suggests that the rationale for providing community assistance to caregiving families might go beyond mere rescue from dire straits to include prevention of distress and promotion of well-being in family caregivers and care-recipients.

The political context in which families care for family members with disabilities has also changed since the dominant paradigm in the study of family care was established. Family caregiving has emerged on the national agenda partly through the formation of national organizations advocating for federal and state legislation aimed at channeling resources to bolster the capacity of families to assist relatives with disabilities. The aging U.S. population has placed an increasing load on the long-term care system, prompting increased attention to the role families can play in efforts to reduce secondary negative effects of disabilities and prevent placements in nursing home and other residential institutions.

As emphasized in this volume, maintaining the current disciplinary "silos" in family research results in lost opportunities. Presently, journals, professional associations, and research communities are separate, determined largely by the disability category or age of the care receivers. People who are elderly are studied by gerontologists who publish in journals devoted exclusively to studies of this group. Similarly, there is a distinctive set of journals and professional associations concerned about individuals with intellectual disabilities. We argue in this volume that much can be gained by making the walls between disciplines more permeable. Theories which can transcend specific disability groups foster such cross fertilization.

In a similar vein, growing cultural diversity in the U.S. poses challenges to the dominant stress and coping paradigm. Some families emigrating from Asia, Africa, and Latin America hold concepts of family, disability, and help giving that differ substantially from those of the Euro-American majority. Thus theories that can provide useful ways of thinking about caregiving in widely diverse cultural contexts across diverse family structures are also needed.

Models of professional-client relationships have also called into question previous beliefs about professional dominance in helping relationships and about the role of bureaucracy in help-giving organizations. For example, the way power and control of resources for caregiving families has been held by bureaucratic systems of care have been questioned. As an alternative to top down control, there has been a movement to establish ways for families to be responsible for determining how to best use public funds for supporting their capacity to help family members with disabilities. Several authors have suggested that transferring control and resources directly to consumers of services will require a new understanding of how professionals provide help. There is also a need to establish what kinds of help should be made available and at what point in time. Early forms of family assistance for family caregiving were primarily concerned with a residual group of families receiving assistance only after their capacity to provide care has broken down. More recent public policy and advocacy efforts have begun to have a preventative focus aimed at providing supports to prevent failure of family care.

Each of the four chapters in the first section of this volume makes contributions toward relevant and widely applicable approaches to family caregiving in our changing society. Brief summaries of the major themes of these chapters follow.

Singer, Biegel, and Ethridge - Toward A Cross Disability View of Family Support for Caregiving Families

Family members provide the majority of care for individuals with disabilities in the U.S. A variety of informal and formal support services have been developed to help reduce the emotional, financial and physical costs of caregiving by these caregivers. These supports, however, are minimal compared to the extent of the need for community resources to bolster the family caregiving role. As Singer, Biegel, and Ethridge discuss in this chapter, much of caregiving research, practice and policy is disease or disability specific. The authors discuss the limitations of this approach, which often amounts to "re-inventing the wheel." Thus, conceptual frameworks, programs and policies often fail to build on knowledge learned about caregiving with one chronic illness, such as Alzheimer's disease, that might be applied to another, such as Schizophrenia.

Singer, Biegel, and Ethridge argue that a cross-categorical framework is needed to enhance caregiving research, practice, and policy. Such an approach would be based on a functional analysis of disability, family caregiving, and the kinds of supports that caregivers require. Across chronic conditions, caregivers who provide the highest levels of care experience similar problems. In addition, a review of the research on caregiver burden in categorical research suggests that many functions that caregivers perform are likely to be more similar across conditions than different. Thus, the authors believe that, given the commonalities inherent in family caregiving regardless of why a care recipient needs assistance, ideas developed in one categorical area are likely to be equally helpful in others. Further, recent research suggests that family caregiving can be associated with positive impacts on the family under the right conditions. The authors provide examples from theory (contribution of feminist perspectives), program design (consumer-directed care) and research (effectiveness of caregiver support programs) that demonstrate the value and usefulness of their cross-categorical framework.

Dunst and Trivette - Capacity-Building Family-Systems Intervention Practices

As Dunst and Trivette indicate, most early childhood initiatives during the 1960's to the 1980's were based on the perceived deficits of children, their parents, or their environment. Over a quarter of a century ago, Dunst and Trivette were instrumental in the transformation of deficit-based, child-focused, early intervention programs into strength-based, family-focused, early childhood intervention and family support programs. This chapter describes a revised and updated approach to early intervention and family support originally presented in their 1988 book *Enabling and Empowering Families.*

In assessing their early intervention and family support model twenty years after its original publication, the authors stated that most surprising was the fact that "nearly all the principles and practices have stood the test of time and still have value for guiding early childhood intervention and family support." The updated version of their model's four operational components of family-systems assessment and intervention has been refined based on research and practice. As the authors indicate, the model is implemented by using capacity-building, help-giving practices to identify family concerns and priorities, the supports and resources that can be used to address concerns and priorities, and the use of family member abilities and interests as the skills to obtain supports and resources. The chapter summarizes findings from research syntheses showing the relationship between different components of the family-systems model and parent, family, and child behavior and functioning; future directions for this field are delineated. Although it has been developed and implemented in the field of early intervention for young children, this model is appealing as a possible cross-disability family support framework. The capacity building and strength based approaches, as well as help-giving which empowers caregivers, are all directly applicable to other populations at other life stages.

Kahana, Kahana, Wykle, and Kulle - Marshalling Social Support: A Care-Getting Model for Persons Living With Cancer

In their chapter on care-getting, Kahana, Kahana, Wykle, and Kulle remind us that caregiving is a two way process that involves both the care-recipient's needs and desires as well as those of the caregiver. While the literature has focused primarily on chronic illnesses with the needs and desire of the caregiver, attention also needs to be paid to the care-recipient's needs and desires. In fact, perhaps the term care-recipient is not an appropriate one, as it implies that the role of persons with a chronic illness is just to passively "receive" care, rather than to proactively "get" care. In this chapter, the authors propose a stress-process theory based conceptual framework for understanding how patients living with cancer can be proactive in care-getting.

The authors' model is an extension of their previously articulated proactivity-based model of successful aging. It is designed to demonstrate how patients can play an active role in obtaining and nurturing care in dealing with life-threatening illness in order to maintain a good quality of life while managing a chronic illness. Although the chapter focuses discussion of the model on patients living with cancer, it is also relevant to patients living with other chronic or life-threatening illnesses. For example, in the past few decades in the literature on developmental disabilities, considerable attention has been focused on empowering consumers to direct their own care and on educating children so that they can take charge as adults.

The care-getting model postulates that, in order for individuals to maintain a good quality of life while dealing with physical or emotional impairments of chronic illnesses or while they encounter acute health events, they must adapt proactively by marshaling informal and formal support resources. In this model, stressors impact quality of life outcomes, which are moderated by care-getting adaptations and resources and the receipt of patient responsive informal and formal care. Examples of the moderator variables in the model include dispositions and attitudes (optimism, resourcefulness, religiosity, and spirituality); proactive adaptations (marshaling support, health care advocacy, planning, and use of technology); informal support resources; and formal support resources. In the developmental disabilities arena, researchers have experimentally demonstrated that adolescents with a variety of disabilities can be taught the skills needed to seek social support for attaining self-determined goals and to negotiate assistance.

Epley, Summers, and Turnbull - Characteristics and Trends in Family-Centered Conceptualizations

Family-centered practice has been an important concept of early intervention and early childhood special education for the past thirty years. As Epley, Summers and Turnbull discuss in their chapter, it has in fact become an integral principle that guides the design and delivery of service delivery models. Its principles have now become embedded in public policy, such as the Individuals with Disabilities Education Act.

Epley and colleagues point out that, despite the importance and centrality of family-centered care, there is a lack of consensus in defining family-centered care. Thus, the focus of this conceptual chapter is to examine current definitions of family-centered care in order to determine if a common definition exists and, if so, whether that definition has changed significantly over the past decade. The authors approach this task by conducting a comprehensive review of 63 peer-reviewed journal articles on family-centered practices published between 1996 and 2007 across disciplines (education, social work, and health). In reviewing these articles, the authors' framework focuses on five key elements: family as the unit of attention, family choice, family strengths, family-professional relationship, and individualized family services. The authors found that, though the key elements of family centeredness (i.e., family choice, family strengths, family-professional relationship, and individualized family services) have remained constant, over time, the emphasis has shifted from the family as the unit of attention to family-professional relationship and family choice. The authors recommend that national family organizations and professional organizations across disciplines involved in early intervention/early childhood services should work together to explicate essential elements of family centeredness. This should then be followed by research investigations on how best to prepare early childhood professionals to implement family-centered practice.

Part II: Empirical Research

The social sciences have developed powerful intellectual tools for description, analysis, and evaluation of important social problems and interventions to address them. An ideal motivating much of this social scientific work is the hope that public policy will be shaped not only by the give and take of political action but also by trustworthy knowledge about the nature of problems and the efficacy of tested approaches toward addressing them. One well established finding across the different disciplines and disability foci is that caregiving changes over the life cycle so that it is not only helpful to compare research across disabilities but also across different stages of the lifecycle. The studies in this section ask questions which cut across different disability groups and different stages in the family lifecycle.

The design of services is likely to influence family adaptation over the lifecycle. Over the past decade there has been considerable interest in empowering people with disabilities to direct their support from social agencies. The first chapter in this section illustrates this important trend in an evaluation of a consumer directed care program.

An important determinant of family life, in addition to the stage of the family lifecycle and the nature of a family member's disability, is the make-up of the family. The impacts of caregiving on marriage, divorce, and remarriage have been assumed to be predominantly negative until recently. The second chapter in this section examines the impact of childhood chronic illness on couples and couple relationships. It exemplifies the growing challenge to the stress, burden, and distress model which has predominated.

Finally, regardless of the cause of the care recipient's disability, the life stage and make-up of the family, in our increasingly multi-cultural society understanding caregiving families in light of their cultures is critical. The third chapter in this section illustrates work in this domain, a study of Latino caregivers. Together these studies point to areas of inquiry important for understanding and serving the rapidly growing number of caregiving families in a changing social and intellectual context. Brief summaries of the major themes of each of the three chapters in this section of our book are presented below.

Vinton - Caregivers' Perceptions of a Consumer-Directed Care Program for Adults With Developmental Disabilities

Consumer choice, autonomy, and self-determination are important themes undergirding programs and policies for both persons with disabilities and family members providing care. As Vinton notes in this chapter, consumer-directed support programs' major goal is shifting more authority and responsibility from service providers to consumers and/or their family members. These programs are both national, such as the Cash and Counseling Demonstration and Evaluation Program, as well as State level, such as California's In-Home Support Services or Illinois' Home Based Support Services Program.

Previous research studies focused primarily on program costs and rates of institutionalization. More recently, however, studies have also examined the perceptions of both consumers and family caregivers about these programs. This chapter, using both quantitative and qualitative methods, examines results from a 12 month consumer and care-giver directed pilot program for families with adults with developmental disabilities, implemented in three sites in one southeastern US state. Pre and post surveys of 50 caregivers examined perceptions of choice, goodness of fit of services to consumer's needs, and satisfaction with services and the program. In addition, focus groups were conducted with 44 individuals, including caregivers, consumers, and support coordinators. Findings showed significant pre to post changes in caregivers' perceptions of choice, goodness-of-fit of services to the needs, and satisfaction with the program. Themes from the focus groups identified the program's value in terms of establishing trust in providers, flexibility in service delivery, and relief and respite.

McCoyd, Akincigil, and Paek - Pediatric Disability and Caregiver Separation

Parents who have a child who is born with a disability can experience significantly more stress than parents of children who are not born with a disability. McCoyd and colleagues indicate that, for a number of years practice wisdom equaled the thought that parents who had a child born with a disability were at much higher risk for marital dissolution than other parents. However, previous research results have been equivocal and the studies themselves have a number of methodological limitations. Previous studies have tended to used small, non-representative samples and have generally not focused on the identification of moderating and mediating variables that are protective or challenging to the family caregivers.

To address these limitations of the extant research on this topic, McCoyd and colleagues used a large, nationally representative sample of families who had experience with Supplemental Security Income (National Survey of Supplemental Income Children and Families). The authors' study of 1,123 caregivers explored the impact of family caregiving and burden for children with disabilities on the stability of the caregiver's primary relationship and identified risk or protective factors associated with stability of that relationship. Study findings did not indicate a statistically significant relationship between caregiver burden and marital separation or a statistically significant relationship between higher levels of disability severity and marital separation. Only the instability of the child's condition and extremely higher levels of caregiver burden (the need for respite care and the need for the family to provide more than 48 hours of home health care), were positively associated with relationship separation. Use of a support group was associated with lower levels of relationship dissolution. This study is valuable in part because it not only examines contributors to family distress, but also those variables which enhance family resilience. Again, the question of what formal and informal elements support positive outcomes in family caregiving needs to be asked across disabilities, cultural groups, and lifecycle stages.

Magaña and Ghosh - Latina Mothers Caring for a Son or Daughter with Autism or Schizophrenia: Similarities, Differences, and the Relationship Between Co-Residency and Maternal Well-Being

Latinos represent the largest minority population in the United States and now compose 16% of the total population of the U.S., according to the 2010 Census. In fact, more than half of the growth in the total population of the United States between 2000 and 2010 was due to the increase in the Latino population. Thus, caregiving for this population is an increasingly salient issue. While, as the authors report, a moderate amount of research about Latino caregivers of older adults with dementia and other disabilities has been conducted, there is a gap in the Latino caregiving literature across disability contexts. Such research is needed to help determine how caregiving experiences might be similar or different depending on the diagnosis of the care recipient, as this is important information for guiding the development of interventions for caregivers.

This empirical chapter by Sandy Magaña and Subharati Ghosh focuses on Latina mothers who provide care for their own young or adult children with one of two neurological disorders—autism or schizophrenia. The chapter explores whether maternal depressive symptoms and psychological well-being differ between the two groups of mothers, the predictors of maternal depressive symptoms and psychological well-being for the overall sample, and the relationship between co-residency and maternal well-being. Subjects were 29 Latina mothers with a son or daughter with autism and 33 Latina mothers with a son or daughter with schizophrenia. Key findings demonstrated that mothers of adults with schizophrenia had lower levels of psychological well-being than mothers of youth or adults with autism. The mothers' level of depressive symptomatology did not differ by diagnosis. For the overall sample, mothers who co-resided with their son or daughter had lower levels of depressive symptomatology. The authors discuss the role that cultural values play in maternal responses to the caregiver role.

Part III: Public Policy

Many believe that the scale of the challenges posed by the aging U.S. population and the growth in numbers of citizens with chronic conditions requires a response on a scale that must be addressed through public policy. In a democracy, groups of people motivated by personal and family issues can mobilize to seek help from the government in obtaining resources that otherwise are not available. In C. Wright Mill's famous formulation, personal problems become public issues when groups of people realize that their own problems are shared with many others. Through a process of organizing and advocacy, they become political constituencies. This process has been underway for several decades. Groups such as the National Alliance for the Mentally Ill, the ARC (advocating on behalf of individuals with intellectual disabilities), and the American Association of Retired Persons, as well as a number of other organizations, are focused on the needs of people with many different chronic conditions. More recently, distinctive organizations devoted to caregiving families across disability categories also have emerged on the national level. That is, a constituency focused on the needs of caregiving families in general has entered the public arena at a national level.

For example, the National Respite Coalition has successfully influenced legislation at a national level, providing funds to assist states to develop comprehensive, cross categorical respite care programs.

One key question regarding public policy concerns is which family outcomes are desirable and how to measure them. This is a foundational question that must be settled in order to make progress in evaluating family support policies. Traditional appeals for resources to support family caregiving have emphasized prevention of institutionalization as their rationale and goal. This goal is important because of the fiscal and human costs of institutionalization of people with disabilities. It is, however, an insufficient goal when considering the needs of family caregivers. Theory and research on service philosophy, design, intervention, and evaluation are all important inputs for policy makers and policy implementers.

The two chapters in this section of the book focus on this broader level of analysis about conceptualizing and designing supports to bolster the caregiving capacity of families in the U.S. Brief summaries of the major themes of each chapter are presented below.

Wang and Brown - Family Quality of Life: A Framework for Policy and Social Service Provisions to Support Families of Children With Disabilities

The Quality of Life framework has been widely used in the disability field to guide service delivery and policy in order to enhance outcomes of individuals with disabilities. Over the last two decades, this framework has been extended to families and has been recognized as an important concept in the area of family supports. However, as Wang and Brown point out, few empirical studies, especially in the field of social work, have examined the Family Quality of Life (FQoL) framework. This chapter provides an overview of the conceptualization, measurement and application of FQoL and its value in the context of family supports for families of children with intellectual and developmental disabilities.

The authors state that FQoL has emerged in response to the need for a strengths-based theoretical and conceptual framework that can help guide the development of family-centered approaches to family support. The authors review findings from two separate teams who have worked on the conceptualization of the multi-dimensional concept of FQoL. Wang & Brown review work on the measurement of FQoL, indicating that, although much of the previous research has utilized qualitative measures of FQoL, two different quantitative scales have been developed to measure FQoL—*The Family Quality of Life Scale* and the *Family Quality of Life Survey*. The authors discuss the implications of this work for the field of social work and offer recommendations on how FQoL can be used in practice and service delivery.

Singer, Biegel, and Ethridge - Trends Impacting Public Policy Support for Caregiving Families

A variety of demographic, social, and economic factors have brought the needs of caregiving families to the attention of public policy makers. This chapter by Singer, Biegel, and Ethridge discusses trends, current policy initiatives and challenges for the future. Family caregiving is ubiquitous in American society, with almost one-third of the adult population providing care to a relative or friend with physical or mental disabilities. Though having positive rewards for the caregiver, caregiving can have substantial physical, social and financial costs for the caregiver as well.

The authors suggest that public policy for caregiving can only be understood through the backdrop of cultural and historical values, such as the residual social welfare system in the U.S., a gender bias of unpaid or under-paid caregiving work of women, and the concept of *home* as the preferred place for living a life marked by self-determination and individualism. In reviewing current public policy supports for family caregiving, the authors conclude that policy has been characterized by piecemeal programs of relatively small scope leading to lack of consistency and coordination.

However, the authors point out that support is growing for moving beyond policy fragmentation and incrementalism. This effort has been led by coalitions with shared interests in family support. An example of such efforts is the Lifespan Respite Care Act of 2006, which created national funding streams for States to establish coordinated systems of respite care for families of children and adults with disabilities. The result is a life-span approach rather than age or disease specific approaches to addressing caregiver needs.

Toward A Cross Disability View of Family Support for Caregiving Families

GEORGE H. S. SINGER

Gevirtz Graduate School of Education, University of California, Santa Barbara, California

DAVID E. BIEGEL

Mandell School of Applied Social Sciences, Case Western University, Cleveland, Ohio

BRANDY L. ETHRIDGE

Gevirtz Graduate School of Education, University of California, Santa Barbara, California

Family members provide the majority of care for individuals with disabilities in the United States. There is growing recognition that family caregiving deserves and may require societal support, and evidence-based practices have been established for reducing stress associated with caregiving. A substantial research literature on family support has developed, but researchers, advocates, and professionals have often worked in separate categorical domains such as family support for caregiving for the frail elderly, for individuals with mental illnesses, and for people with developmental disabilities. This article considers the merits of a cross-categorical analysis of family support. Examples of concepts from one domain of family support are applied to other domains to illustrate the potential benefits of a broader exchange of ideas.

This essay considers the prospects for a cross-disability approach to understanding and supporting the caregiving functions of families. This special edition of the *Journal of Family Social Work* and a subsequent edition that will follow within the year are designed to encourage an exchange of ideas about family support across the various categorical discourses that presently characterize research regarding the provision of support for the caregiving functions of families. Caregivers support family members who experience disabilities related to many different physical and cognitive impairments that restrict normal functioning. These disabilities can first become evident at any time, ranging from birth, in the case of children born with some developmental disabilities, to advanced old age, in the case of family caregivers for relatives with dementia. In the United States and Canada, the family is now the main provider of long-term care, even for people with severe disabilities (McKeever, 1996; Pandya, 2005).

Family support refers to a constellation of formal and informal resources designed to promote the benefits and reduce the various social costs of family caregiving for individuals with physical and cognitive impairments. Ideally, the goal of family support is to enhance the quality of life of the caregiving family and the individual who is the care recipient (Wang & Brown, in press). The giving of assistance and support by one family member to another is a regular and usual part of family interactions. Thus, it is in fact a normative and pervasive activity. Caregiving due to chronic illness and disability represents something that, in principle, is not very different from traditional tasks and activities rendered to family members. The difference is that "caregiving" in this situation represents the increment of extraordinary care that goes beyond the bounds of normal or usual care (Biegel, Sales, & Schulz, 1991). For 2 decades, researchers and advocates have argued the case for promotional as well as ameliorative family supports; however, from the point of view of policy makers, the purpose of family support has often been to reduce the long-term fiscal costs of care related to potentially avoidable institutionalization and worsening of disabilities (Arno, Levine, & Memmott, 1999; Dunst & Trivette, in press).

Family caregiving for family members who need assistance with activities required for independent living is one of the most important and enduring functions of families in the United States. It is of such great worth, not only because caregiving can be an expression of some of the most salutary characteristics of people and families, but also because of its extent and the costs of replacing it with formal supports. At least 80% of long-term care in the United States is provided informally by family members or friends (National Alliance for Caregiving and AARP, 2004). Caregiving can tax the financial, physical, and psychological resources of caregivers with resulting emotional and physical distress and, in some cases, mortality (Biegel, Ishler, Katz, & Johnson, 2007; Schulz & Beach, 1999; Witt, Riley, & Coiro, 2003). It ranges from brief intermittent help provided to family members during times of illness or injury to intensive live-in caregiving for family members with the most severe impairments, such as advanced Alzheimer's disease, severe autism, and severe mental illness. Caregiving activities range from hands-on help with the care recipient's activities of daily living (ADL), to vigilance of the care recipient, to advocacy with professional service providers. There is substantial evidence of a direct relationship between the perceived burden of caregiving and both depression and physical illness in caregivers. The association of caregiving with psychological distress exists in family caregivers of elderly people with dementia (Schulz & Martire, 2004), caregivers of children with developmental disabilities (Singer, 2006) and chronic illness (Ireys, Chernoff, DeVet, & Kim, 2001), and family caregivers for people with severe and persistent mental illness (Seltzer, Greenberg, Floyd, Pettee, & Hong, 2001; Townsend, Biegel, Ishler, Wieder, & Rini, 2006). These costs are amplified by the collision of caregiving as a traditional female role and the increasing percentage of women who are single parents and who work full time (Walker, Pratt, & Eddy, 1995). Caregiver distress is also exacerbated by the many problems of poverty and by a pileup of stressors in a family (Singer, Goldberg-Hamblin, Peckham-Hardin, Barry, & Santarelli, 2002). However, it is increasingly evident from research that it is a mistake to solely view family caregiving as a stressor because there are potentially uplifts and benefits of family caregiving, not only to the care recipients, but also to the caregivers (Hastings & Taunt, 2002; Greenberg, Greenley, & Benedict, 1994; Walker et al., 1995). Consequently, support for caregiving families ought to be aimed at not only reducing stress and ameliorating distress but also at promoting the potential positive benefits to the caregiver and care receiver.

An estimate of the number of people providing informal care to a family member with a disability is derived from the National Survey of Family Households (National Alliance for Caregiving and AARP, 2004). Caregivers were defined as individuals over the age of 19 who provided care to a relative who had a disability or serious illness. Based on this definition, an estimated 15.9% of adult men and women in the United States served as caregivers, roughly 48 million people in 2007. When the age range of caregivers was expanded to include 18-year-olds, a recent survey of caregivers for elderly family members found an even higher percentage: 22% of all households in the United States included a family caregiver (Pandya, 2005). Thus, close to 20% of the U.S. population helps a relative who experiences a malady or disability on a regular basis for an average of eight hours per week or more. Roughly one in five of these family caregivers provides support for 40 hours a week or more (National Alliance for Caregivers and AARP, 2004). In an analysis of the economic value of informal caregiving, Arno et al. (1999) estimated that annual substitution costs of professional services for the informal care families provide would range from $115 billion to $268 billion, depending on the estimated pay rate. Although informal care is unpaid, it entrains social costs, which are of growing concern as the population in the United States ages and the prevalence of chronic illnesses and disabilities grows.

CAREGIVING TRENDS

Several trends have simultaneously increased the caregiving load in the United States while reducing the traditional capacity of families to provide support. Deinstitutionalization has led to growth in the numbers of individuals with mental impairments who require monitoring and support from family members in the community. Family members include people with severe mental illnesses and individuals with cognitive impairments such as intellectual disabilities and autism. Most individuals with mental retardation live with their families of origin well into middle age (Fujiura, 1998), and a child's severe mental illness can continue to impact the family of origin lifelong (Seltzer et al., 2001). Changes in health care reimbursement and medical technology have increased responsibilities of family caregivers. Not only are family members who are hospitalized experiencing shorter hospital stays, but at the same time, advances in medical technology have increased the numbers of family members who are being sent home to family caregivers who must administer drugs and monitor the patient's medical regime.

Severe chronic illnesses are more prevalent than they were prior to the emergence of antibiotics and hygienic public health measures. Many formerly short-term fatal physical illnesses are now chronic conditions that may limit daily activities and require ongoing monitoring and can necessitate assistance with common activities, such as traumatic brain injury, HIV/AIDS, several forms of cancer, severe heart disease, and chronic obstructive pulmonary disease. Chronic illness has become more common in childhood, as have impairments associated with autism disorder (Center for Disease Control, 2008; Newacheck, Kim, Blumberg, & Rising, 2008). At the other end of the age span, approximately 35% of individuals who require more intensive support with ADL and independent activities of daily living (IADL's) were people over the age of 65 in 1997, and this population is growing dramatically (Kennedy, LaPlante, & Kaye, 1997). The fastest growing subgroup within the aging population is made up of individuals 85 years and older (Federal Interagency Forum on Aging-Related Statistics, 2008). In advanced old age, chronic mental and physical conditions are almost inevitable and regular need for some assistance is common. The percentage of elderly people 85 and older is expected to grow by roughly 400% by the middle of the 21st century (Federal Interagency Forum on Aging-Related Statistics, 2008). These trends have and will continue to place unprecedented demands on the caregiving capacity of families.

The demand for caregiving has increased, not only because of the aging of the population, but also from dramatic changes in the prevalence of chronic illness. The nature of illness has evolved dramatically since the discovery of antibiotics in the early 20th century. The most common serious illnesses traditionally lasted a short time, often ending in death. Since the early 20th century, the prevalence of serious acute illness has waned and the prevalence of chronic illness greatly increased. Many illnesses that were usually brief and often fatal are now chronic, including some forms of cancer, HIV, cystic fibrosis, and congestive heart disease. Severe illnesses that are not fatal but debilitating over a long duration are increasingly common, including arthritis, heart failure, and chronic pulmonary disorders. Nearly 25% of people aged 65 and older were functionally disabled in 1999, and by the year 2040, this number is expected to increase dramatically as the numbers of people over 60 expands (U.S. Census Bureau, 2008).

Caregiving is no longer primarily needed for a few weeks or months during a loved one's acute illness. Instead, the need for assistance with daily living commonly lasts for years (Kunkel & Applebaum, 1999). The average family caregiver for an elderly relative provides care for 4.3 years (National Alliance on Caregiving and AARP, 2004). In the case of individuals with moderate and severe intellectual disabilities (ID), help from family members may last a lifetime, with the caregiving role transferred from parents in late life to siblings (Seltzer & Kraus, 2001). The majority of adults with ID, an estimated 60%, live with their parents well into the parents' old age (Fujiura, 1998; Seltzer & Kraus, 2001). Other long-lasting conditions such as severe and persistent mental illnesses, for example, schizophrenia, typically occur in late adolescence or early adulthood and may persist for a number of years; thus, caregiving by parents can extend for a significant period of years.

At the same time that the need for family caregiving is increasing, the demographic makeup of families has undergone extensive change. Historically, families have grown smaller over the past century, leaving fewer individuals available to provide care. In 1900, the average household had 4.6 family members, compared with an average of 2.6 in 1990 (U.S Census Bureau, 1996). Traditionally, caregiving was primarily carried out by women. In 2005, the typical caregiver was a 46-year-old woman who delivered more than 20 hours of care weekly to her mother (Pandya, 2005). Although 40% of caregivers are men, on average they provide less care for shorter duration than women (National Alliance for Caregivers and AARP, 2004).

Feminism has challenged the assumption that women, as a matter of course, should take on the main duties of caregiving (Hooyman & Gonyea, 1995). Although 40% of family caregivers are men, women remain the primary caregivers and constitute a kind of shadow workforce for the health care industry (Bookman & Harington, 2007; Walker et al., 1995). The majority of men involved with caregiving provide help for relatives with lower levels of need and provide more care management than hands-on care. Among caregivers of elderly relatives, women make up 51% of caregivers for individuals requiring the least amount of care, defined as fewer than eight hours a week, compared to 71% who care for relatives who need full-time care, including help with basic ADL. An additional strain arises from conflicts between caregiving that may be necessary at any time of the day and employment. A majority of caregivers for the elderly ages 18 to 64 are employed full or part time (National Alliance for Caregiving and AARP, 2004). It is no longer taken for granted that mothers and daughters should be expected to sacrifice careers and other life goals to care for relatives with disabilities, although such sacrifices are quite common when other care arrangements are not affordable or acceptable.

Family caregiving impacts employment in ways that create a need for community supports designed to reduce the number or work hours caregivers miss (MetLife Mature Market Institute and National Alliance for Caregiving, 2006). Businesses lose an estimated $17 to $34 billion from the cost of employees who must give up work hours to attend to caregiving responsibilities (MetLife, 2006). Studies of employed men and women caregivers have conflicting findings about whether or not employment adds to their stress or buffers it (Edwards, Zarit, Stevens, & Townsend, 2002). Edwards et al. found that caregivers who reported conflicts on the job had the highest levels of strain related to caregiving. In one large study, stress was the greatest for employed caregivers who were responsible for more than one care recipient, as is the case of women who were caring for elderly family members and children with chronic illnesses or disabilities (Neal, Chapman, Ingersoll-Dayton, & Emlen, 1993).

FUNCTIONAL AND CATEGORICAL VIEWS OF FAMILY SUPPORT AND CAREGIVING

There is a paradox in the ways that family support and family caregiving are currently conceptualized. On one hand, the current taxonomy of caregiving for vulnerable family members is defined in a noncategorical manner by functionality. On the other hand, the great majority of policies, practices, and research on family support are constructed along categorical lines, usually based on medical diagnostic categories. For example, there are different professional journals and associations that presently include family support as part of their areas of concern; these include separate approaches for caregiving families falling into each of the following broad disability categories: chronic illnesses, developmental disabilities, mental illness, and the conditions associated with old age. Gerontologists focus on caregivers of elderly family members; psychologists, psychiatrists, and social workers focus on the families of individuals with mental illness, though families are often excluded from the mental health treatment process. Still, other professionals, pediatricians and nurses, focus their work on children with chronic illnesses and their families.

This approach has been heavily influenced by medicine, with its emphasis on the diagnosis and treatment of discrete diseases and with its specializations clustered around different anatomical systems. Medicalization has brought with it the virtues of specialization in which in-depth knowledge can be developed in a discrete field of focus. However, it also may obscure commonalities that may be important for public policy, research pertaining to the design and testing of service systems, the training of professionals, and for building a sense of political solidarity around a public agenda focusing on community assistance to bolster the caregiving capacities of families. By defining nonmedical problems a priori in medical language, medicalization also risks obscuring the social trends and political motives that are shaping the growth of family home caregiving in the United States and the resultant growing need for family support. There are, however, some disciplines that are better suited by their basic design and mission to address the needs of people with functional limitations and their caregiving families in a more generic way; social work is particularly appropriate for this role.

A cross-categorical conceptualization of family support is based on a functional analysis of disability as well as family caregiving and kinds of supports caregivers require. Caregiving and the functioning of the care receiver are, of course, closely linked and can both be described in terms of the impact of the illness or impairment on common activities. The Americans with Disability Act (ADA; U.S. Department of Justice, 2008) and Section 504 of the Rehabilitation Act define disability functionally (Yell, 2006). A U.S. citizen is eligible for protection under these laws if they experience a physical or mental impairment that substantially limits one or more major life activities. These activities are defined in the ADA as caring for one's self, performing manual tasks, walking, seeing, hearing, speaking, breathing, learning, and working (ADA, 1990). The National Association of Caregivers and the AARP (2004) define the level of need that a family caregiver must meet by the number of caregiving activities they carry out and the amount of time devoted to them. A perusal of measures of caregiver burden that have been developed in categorical research suggests that many functions that caregivers perform are likely to be more the same across conditions than different. These include balancing work and caregiving demands, providing transportation, shopping for the care receiver, monitoring his or her health and well-being, interceding with bureaucracies, communicating with various professionals, giving medicine, preparing meals, helping with personal hygiene, managing their finances, and managing problem behavior (Biegel et al., 1991; Novak & Guest, 1989).

The kinds of problems that caregivers experience are also similar among caregivers who provide the highest levels of care. These problems include elevated levels of mental health problems, particularly depression, and a higher prevalence of physical illness (National Alliance for Caregivers and AARP, 2004; Witt et al., 2003). Across chronic illnesses of adults, perceived care recipient behavioral problems are the strongest predictor of caregiver burden (Biegel et al., 1991). When examined from a functional perspective, there appear to be many commonalities to family caregiving regardless of the cause of the care recipient's impairments (Biegel et al., 1991). For example, advocates for caregivers of children with developmental disabilities and other advocates for caregivers of family members with dementia have both successfully pushed for federal and state support for respite care. The recently enacted National Caregivers Program (Older Americans Act, 2000) encourages states to develop interagency cooperation between respite care programs across populations. Although most programs for supporting caregiving families are mandated at the state level, several federal laws also create an entitlement for some limited services (Ethridge & Singer, 2009). These laws demonstrate a convergence at the public policy level on similar needs across disability categories.

DIFFERENCE AND SAMENESS NEEDS TO BE RECOGNIZED

It is our purpose here to point out some of the commonalities inherent in family caregiving regardless of why a care recipient needs assistance and to illustrate some of the ideas developed in one categorical area but are likely to be equally helpful in others. Before proceeding to identify areas of sameness and potential benefits of a functional and noncategorical approach, we need to acknowledge that the kinds of differentiation that presently typify the study of family caregiving are based in very real differences between the conditions that cause a family member to need unusual levels of help, and in some instances there are equally important differences in the caregivers. Developmental disability and dementia, for example, occur at opposite ends of the life span. Families of children with developmental disabilities are likely to begin their roles as caregivers when the families are in an early stage of the life cycle, whereas the typical caregiver for elderly family members with dementia are either same-age spouses or middle-aged daughters (National Alliance for Caregivers, 2004). Disability categories also vary, in some cases, according to the main social institutions and professions that define them. A family caring for a family member with schizophrenia is likely to need access to psychiatrists and mental health case managers, many of whom are social workers, and to acquire the language and ways of thinking specific to the mental health professions. By contrast, the parents of a child with autism may primarily rely on special educators and behavioral psychologists for technical advice on caregiving.

Disease entities also vary in the kinds of associated impairments, so that family members with severe arthritis may need home modifications to make their homes accessible to a wheelchair, whereas an adult with mental retardation may need skills instruction on independent living skills. Diseases vary also in whether they are stable or degenerative, terminal or chronic. Conditions further differ by the extent to which they are stigmatized by the surrounding society; mental retardation or mental illness may have more negative associations for the public than advanced old age (Link, Mirotznik, & Cullen, 1991). Despite these and many other real differences, there are also real costs in only seeing these differences and organizing scholarship and the professions around discrete disease entities or ages. Two major ways that family caregiving is similar regardless of the disability of the care receiver are the kinds of supports families need and the potential financial, social, and emotional costs of family caregiving.

Advocates have successfully championed federal and state policies at least at a nascent level to provide some forms of support to some caregiving families, primarily to reduce caregiver burden, stress, and distress while reducing the use of expensive institutional services for family members with disabilities. Federal statutes addressing the needs of several different vulnerable populations mandate some forms of family support for caregivers, although these are in several cases secondary to the main purposes of the laws. These laws are designed to build services commonly delivered by social workers, including case management, information and referral services, support groups, and counseling for family caregivers. Family support for caregivers is relatively new, and the availability of services and benefits varies greatly with the locale, the degree to which a service system has been developed for a particular chronic condition, and the accessibility of the supports that have been established. The degree to which support systems have been established varies with the amount of time the mandates have been in place and the extent to which resources have been allocated to implement them. The longest standing mandate for federal assistance is in the Social Security Income Disability Act, which gives funds to low-income families of individuals with designated disabilities. Early intervention services for children with developmental disabilities have been designed by law to be family centered since 1985. Although implementation has often been difficult, parent satisfaction with the services has been high (McWilliam et al., 1995; Romer & Umbreit, 1998). The service system for people with intellectual disabilities through the full life cycle is one of the most developed for any vulnerable population. However, expenditures for family support for families of individuals with developmental disabilities who reside at home make up less than 5% of the funds allocated for services for this population (Braddock, 2002), despite the fact that approximately 60% of these individuals reside with their parents well into the care receivers' middle age and the caregiver's old age. Although federal mandates are extremely important for establishing uniform policies and creating funding streams for services, most support services are created and funded in varying degrees by the states. An example of the variability in and the limited implementation of family support policy and practices can be seen in data on an index of six practices advocated by the National Alliance for the Mentally Ill (NAMI) that are widely recognized as valuable and essential for family support. On average, the 51 states and territories evaluated by NAMI fell short of full implementation on all of these items. Five of these goals are held in common by advocates across the three other disability groups: (a) ready access via the Internet and telephone to family-friendly, culturally competent information and referral services, (b) family participation in the monitoring of service quality, (c) family support groups, (d) psychoeducation, and (e) state financial and logistic support to family-to-family self-help programs. NAMI's survey of the quality of care for people with mental illness in the United States found that these goals were rarely realized (NAMI, 2006). By contrast, early intervention services for families of children with developmental delays or disabilities are delivered by a much more developed service system and consumer satisfaction is much higher than for families of people with serious mental illness (Bailey, Hebbeler, Scarborough, & Sangeeta, 2004).

DISCIPLINARY BOUNDARIES IN RESEARCH ON FAMILY SUPPORT

Research, advocacy, and social services for people with disabilities have generally been organized around a typology of physical and cognitive impairments designated by medical diagnostic categories. In the literature on family caregiving, separate lines of work are grouped by the broad categories of chronic physical illnesses, mental illnesses, developmental disabilities, and conditions arising in old age. These general categories are further divided into more specialized conditions so that, for example, there is a literature on family caregiving for people with dementia as distinguished from research on caregiving for elderly people with other physical conditions, a literature on parents of children with autism separate from studies of parents of children with mental retardation, and distinctive literatures on family caring for cancer patients and people with HIV/AIDS. Such differentiations of literature may lead to a reinventing of the wheel with researchers, advocates, and policy makers not being aware of potential commonalities for interventions across problems and illnesses. There is reason to question a sole focus on this categorical approach when considering family caregiving and family support. The functions that families perform and the nature of the stressors, uplifts, and needs for support have important common features regardless of the specific disability category of concern. One important task for researchers and policy makers is to identify which family functions are the same across categories and could benefit from noncategorical forms of support and which are different by virtue of the unique characteristics of diagnostic conditions and thus require special expertise in supporting families with unique clusters of needs.

When considered functionally, many common aspects of caregiving are shared across categories. This commonality is driven largely by the nature of the tasks, routines, and functions that families typically perform for their members, including, at the most general level, the provision of food, shelter, and clothing; provision of emotional and informational support; and shopping and meal preparation. Further, they include transportation to appointments, making of arrangements to deal with unexpected demands and emergencies, leisure and recreation activities, monitoring of health and emotional status, linkage to the community, and bureaucratic mediation such as advocating for needed programs and services for their family members (Kennedy et al., 1997).

Meeting the needs of family members with disabilities entails work. When families cooperate as a team to provide support to their members with disabilities, the health and well-being of the primary caregiver is better and outcomes from people with disabilities are improved (Caruth, Tate, Moffett, & Hill, 1997; Wallander, Varni, Babani, Heatger, & Wilcox, 1989). Family support involves the provision of resources from professionals and service agencies that help families perform these necessary caregiving functions. It also includes helping caregivers attain access to generic social supports already available in the community by linking them, for example, to a church group or an ongoing recreation program.

With some notable exceptions—such as Biegel & Schulz's Family Caregiver Applications Series published by Sage in the 1990s; Singer, Powers, and Olson's work (1996); and a review of the literature on family-centered services across fields (Allen & Petr, 1996)—there has been little scholarly work based on the similar functions that family caregivers perform and the forms of support they need regardless of the diagnostic category applied to family members who require care. The cost of this kind of balkanization of research and advocacy is that important ideas and findings that might be helpful for understanding family support and for promoting new public policy initiatives are walled off from groups that could benefit from the cross-fertilization of ideas. There have been some important examples of this kind of cross-disciplinary analysis. At a definitional level, functional descriptions of disabilities centering around the concepts of ADL and IADL cut across categories and point to the level of care that families are required to provide and, by extrapolation, the kinds of support caregivers are likely to need (Jagger, Antony, Spiers, & Clarke, 2001).

In the psychology literature, there are at least two general forms of interventions for caregivers that have been effective across disability categories. Researchers treating the problem behaviors in individuals with developmental disabilities, people with traumatic brain injury, and elderly people with dementia have taught caregivers the same behavior management methods based on ideas from the discipline of applied behavior analysis (Carnevale, Anselmi, Busicio, & Millis, 2002; Cooper, Heron, & Heward, 2007; Losada, Izal, Perez-Rojo, & Montorio, 2007; Stock & Milan, 1993). Similarly, psychoeducational interventions for caregivers have been effective with family caregivers for children with developmental disabilities (Singer, Ethridge, & Aldana, 2007), people with Alzheimer's disease

(Gallagher-Thompson, & Coon, 2007), and adults with schizophrenia (Biegel, Robinson, & Kennedy, 2000; Lefley, in press). These similar approaches suggest that generic in-home behavioral services and cognitive-behavioral therapeutic services might be an important source of noncategorical support for caregivers of family members with challenging behavior regardless of its etiology.

POTENTIAL FOR CROSS-FERTILIZATION OF CONCEPTS ABOUT FAMILY SUPPORT

This special edition of the *Journal of Family Social Work* and a subsequent second edition aim to promote an exchange of theories and research findings that have a wide applicability across disability categories. The remainder of this article presents three examples of potentially transportable concepts and their empirical bases. The aim is to illustrate the potential benefits of exchanges of ideas and data across traditional disciplinary boundaries. We have selected examples from three levels of analysis: (a) theory, (b) intervention research, and (c) public policy.

Theory: The Contribution of Feminist Perspectives

Feminist scholars have influenced frameworks for mapping key aspects of family caregiving (Fox & Murry, 2000). Authors writing from a feminist stance were among the first to call attention to the family caregiver role, the way it has been undervalued historically, and the way that gender influences the social construction of household divisions of labor (Boserup, 1970; Oakley, 1974; Ruddick, 1989). The majority of family caregiving is provided by women; recent data indicates a growing role for men, but roughly 60% of caregivers for elderly family members are middle-aged females, usually daughters (Pandya, 2005). The mother–daughter relationship has been highlighted in studies influenced by feminist thought. *Attentive love* (Ruddick, 1989) is a construct originally derived from an analysis of maternal thinking as situated in the practices of parenting. Ruddick described attentive love as "a conceptual scheme—a vocabulary and logic of connections—through which they (mothers) order and express the facts and values of their practice" (Ruddick, 1982, p. 77, cited in McGraw & Walker, 1992, p. 284–285). Attentive love, according to Ruddick, enables a woman to realistically understand her children while caring intensely about them. Her efforts focus on meeting three demands that are often in conflict: the need for protection to preserve the life of the child, the need for nurturance to foster competence and lead the child over time to grow beyond dependence, and the need to ensure the child meets the surrounding culture's standard for becoming a productive contributor to society. Researchers have used this framework to examine the thinking embedded in the caregiving practices of middle-aged daughters supporting their elderly mothers (Allan & Walker, 1992; McGraw & Walker, 2004). Based on interviews with 29 caregiving daughters, they identified examples of situated cognition aligned with Ruddick's framework. For example, a middle-aged daughter explained how she made decisions about balancing protectiveness with promoting autonomy when grocery shopping with her mother who had severe arthritis. "I take my mother grocery shopping. She pushes the cart and I run up and down the aisles" (McGraw & Walker, 1992, p. 287). Such decisions are inseparable from their lived context; that is, attentive love is a form of praxis. The concept of attentive love has not been utilized in research on parents of children with disabilities or family caregivers for individuals who are not elderly but experience chronic physical or mental illnesses.

The theory of attentive love appears to be directly transferable to the study of parenting children with disabilities. Undoubtedly, parents of these children think in action about ways to balance protection with promoting independence. These decisions may be a key to the development of a sense of self-determination in young adults with disabilities. Powers, Singer, and Todis (1996) interviewed successful adults with neuromotor disorders who were living independently, meaningfully employed, and who considered themselves to be happy and in charge of their own lives. When asked to describe the origin of their sense of competence, these adults almost uniformly cited the ways that their parents held them to the same standards as their typically developing siblings, while also making accommodations for their disabilities. A graduate student who had polio as a child described the way in which he was expected to do household chores. He was required to do chores for the same length of time as his non-disabled brothers, but his parents assigned tasks that could be done from his wheelchair. His brothers were assigned chores such as mowing the lawn, while he was asked to help with household tasks. He quoted his parents as telling him, "Don't expect anything special. There are some things you'll just have to do differently." The first sentence seems to be a statement from parental situated cognition about nurturing independence, while the second statement would appear to be a reflection of realistic thinking about accommodation, perhaps a form of protective parenting. That is, the balancing of sometimes conflicting demands is likely to be a common feature of everyday thought and practice in families of children with disabilities. Another young man with severe cerebral palsy described the way his father enlisted him to help with outdoor work like stacking firewood. His father built a "kiddy car" that let him position himself so that he could contribute to the work. "[My father] couldn't keep me out of the woodpile. I stacked it with my dad. I did it with one hand" (Powers et al., 1996, p. 80). The attentive love framework might be very useful in pointing out and making sense of the way parents structure daily activities for their disabled children. Similarly, an idea derived from the study of parents of children with developmental delays is likely to be very useful for making sense of how best to support families caring for adults with physical and mental impairments.

Theory: Accounting for Cultural Difference in Daily Accommodations

The second example of a theoretical construct that we believe is transportable and potentially very useful to practitioners of family support is the concept of *sustainable accommodations to daily family routines* (Gallimore, Weisner, Kaufman, & Bernheimer, 1989). It may be very helpful in designing the delivery of family support in a multicultural context. Keogh, Bernheimer, Gallimore, and Weisner (1998) reported findings from a longitudinal study of 103 families of children with developmental delays over a period of several years. These families resided in the greater Los Angeles area and included parents from ethnic and linguistic minority groups as well as different socioeconomic status (SES) levels. Contemporary Los Angeles is a mélange of cultures, and any social worker or social scientist who practices there must deal with the challenges posed by cultural, social class, and linguistic differences. Gallimore and Weisner are educational anthropologists who developed an interview format based on dimensions of family life derived from studies of childrearing across many different cultures. As anthropologists they were attuned to the details of daily routines as enacted by family members. By examining activity contexts (e.g., mealtimes, bedtime, leisure times), they were able to highlight the ways that families worked to preserve the most valued features of their daily routines while also modifying them to meet the needs of their children with disabilities (Gallimore et al., 1989).

The construct, *sustainable accommodations*, is made of three ideas. First, it assumes that much of family life is built around predictable daily routines in which families enact their scripts, values, and goals. The unit of analysis is these routines. Second, they assume that family routines for the most part reflect the practices from parents' cultures of origin and that parents actively try to preserve these routines in their accustomed form. For example, many middle-class Anglo families try to have a family dinner routine in which all family members sit down together with talk about the day as part of the routine. Such routines need to be modified sometimes to meet the caregiving needs of family members with disabilities. For example, a child with a severe neuromotor disorder may need to be spoon fed pureed food. A parent might chose to begin feeding this child before the rest of the family sits down to mealtime, and much of her talk and attention may be directed at the disabled child's eating. She is likely to also try to preserve valued features of the mealtime routine. For example, she may still prepare the food for the other family members, join intermittently in the conversation, and direct the other children to help with cleaning up. Third, to the extent that the mother can maintain this altered routine without unacceptable levels of stress or loss of valued aspects of the routine, the accommodation is sustainable. With this construct in mind, family support can be seen, in part, as efforts to assist families to sustain valued routines. For example, a caseworker might identify the contribution an occupational or physical therapist might make in helping the child to participate more actively in feeding himself. Provision of this support would both benefit the child and help the parent to maintain an important routine. It seems very likely that the idea of sustainable accommodations would be useful in research on caregiving and family support for other populations.

Design of Family Support Services: Consumer-Directed Care

Our third example of a cross-disability construct comes from recent experiments in the design of support services for people with disabilities and their families. A number of initiatives in the United States and Europe have emphasized a cluster of design features that attempt to maximize the autonomy of the care recipients and their families (Powers, Sowers, & Singer, 2006). Family support programs have been impacted by a larger movement for more consumer control in the design and delivery of social services. In the United States, advocates for people with disabilities and their families have asserted their preference for a system of support based more on respect for autonomy, capacity building, and consumer control than more traditional systems that have emphasized paternalistic benevolence, professional expertise, and agency control over allocation of resources and design of services. A central difference between these relatively recent programs and more traditional ones is the nature of the relationship between professionals and service recipients. Turnbull, Turbiville, and Turnbull (2000) characterized traditional hierarchical relationships between professionals and families as *power-over*, as compared to *power-through*, relationships in which the professional becomes an agent for helping the customers to achieve their goals. They emphasize individualized service planning in which the recipients are viewed as customers who are given a great deal of leeway in how they spend cash assistance. Autonomous access to deploying social benefits is gradually being extended to groups of people and their surrogates (usually family members) who previously were thought to be incapable of directing their own services including people with cognitive disabilities. Powers et al. (2006) described this trend in the following way: "Models are being developed that avoid the oversimplified notion that service users are either autonomous or nonautonomous, permitting both collaborative direction of services by individuals and trusted others, and delegated autonomy to surrogates." (p. 67)

Support programs vary on a continuum from almost complete laissez-faire (the agency sends a check to the caregiver) to complete agency control of how services are designed and allocated. Newer service models include (a) direct cash payments to care recipients or family caregivers with some counseling to recipients who are responsible for all aspects of service management, (b) fiscal intermediary programs in which families control the use of funds and the hiring and management of service providers while the intermediary takes care of bookkeeping, payroll, paying taxes, and other administrative tasks, (c) supportive intermediary programs that give help with service coordination, brokering supports, or screening and training care providers, (d) self-directed case management programs in which agencies retain control over funds and services but the consumers are actively engaged in planning and decision making, and (e) spectrum programs in which customers chose from any of the above options (Powers et al., 2006; Velgouse & Dize, 2000).

These consumer-directed service models are all designed with the idea that intervention should empower caregivers and build their capacity to assist other family members while maintaining their own health and well-being. A fundamental element of these service designs is the commitment to establishing more equitable partnerships between caregivers and professionals. These relationships are meant to be based on mutual trust and reciprocity, so that caregivers are recognized as experts in their own right and as contributors to achieving the goals that the professionals and family member share. Researchers have examined the constituent parts of parent–professional partnerships in early intervention and public school programs for children with developmental disabilities (Blue-Banning, Summers, Frankland, Nelson, & Beegle, 2004). Based on focus groups with professionals and parents who had established effective working relationships, they were able to identify common characteristics of productive partnerships. For example, parents reported their appreciation of professionals who were skilled enough to be effective, to "make things happen," but who were also willing to learn from parents and to admit when they did not know something. A caveat was that if professionals admitted to not knowing something, then they needed to find ways to learn it and inform parents of the new information or skills they acquired.

In this issue, Dunst and Trivette (2008) stress the central importance of the way in which helpgiving is delivered. In a recent meta-analysis, they presented evidence from over 40 studies of family–professional relationships in programs for young children with disabilities (Dunst, Trivette, & Hamby, 2007). Their synthesis of the literature indicated that professional helpgiving was most effective when it took two forms, *relational helpgiving* and *participatory helpgiving*. The former consisted of "practices typically associated with good clinical practice (e.g., active listening, compassion, empathy, and respect)" (Dunst et al., 2007, p. 370). The second characteristic of effective helpgiving consisted of flexible and individualized assistance that was responsive to family needs and that engaged parents as both informed decision makers and as active participants in achieving their goals (Dunst et al.). Again, these forms of helpgiving contrast with the traditional medical model in which the professional dispenses expert knowledge while focusing on the help recipient's pathology.

Effectiveness of Programs That Support Family Caregivers

Evaluations of family support programs have been promising. In recent years, researchers have compiled meta-analytic syntheses as well a narrative literature reviews to characterize groups of studies regarding supportive interventions for parents of children with developmental disabilities (Singer, Ethridge, & Aldana, 2007), for family caregivers of older adults (Sorenson, Pinquart, & Duberstein, 2002), elderly people with dementia (Gallagher-Thompson & Coon, 2007), and caregivers of adults with mental illnesses (Biegel et al., 2000). While there are some interventions that are uniquely designed for a specific population, a striking finding in comparing these studies is the similarity in effective treatment approaches. Across conditions, psychoeducational interventions were generally effective, especially longer term treatments. These interventions were usually delivered in groups, although telephone and Internet treatments have also been effective. They provided information on the care receivers' conditions and needs and instruction of coping skills such as problem solving, relaxation training, and increasing pleasant activities (Dixon et al., 2001; Gallagher-Thompson & Coon, 2007). Psychoeducation, including coping skills derived from cognitive behavioral treatments, was also effective across caregivers of people with developmental disabilities and individuals with mental illnesses (Biegel et al., 2000; Lefley, in press; Lozada, Izal, Perez-Rojo, & Montorio, 2007; Singer, Ethridge, & Aldana, 2007).

Interventions to help families caring for a family member with schizophrenia have also shown considerable effects since there are now evidence-based practices in this area (MacFarlane, Dixon, Lukens, & Lucksted, 2007; Lefley, in press). Several studies have shown that family support interventions have been as effective as medication in reducing hospital recidivism for people with schizophrenia (Dixon et al., 2001). There can be little doubt that family support can bolster the caregiving capacity of many families.

In this issue of the *Journal of Family Social Work,* we have invited authors working in different family support fields to contribute conceptual articles that explain ideas that may be more widely applicable across categories. Dunst and Trivette review the evolution of a model for supporting young families of children with disabilities. Their model is thoroughly developed and has considerable empirical support. Their analysis of effective ways to help families should have a broad audience. The article by Wang and Brown similarly comes from work in the developmental disabilities field, but it is a concept that can be readily transferred to other family caregiving populations. They report on the theory behind the development of new measures of family quality of life that are intended as a way to gauge the effect of social policies and interventions aimed at families of individuals with special needs. Again, the concepts here are readily applicable across populations. The article by Kahana et al. comes from a large study of elderly individuals who receive care. Here the focus is on what it means to be a care recipient and the implications for how families might best assist elderly family members. The emphasis on care receiving represents an interesting shift in the focus of research and one population of people with need for caregiving, and, again, the idea may serve as a spark for new work in other fields. In summary, in this and a subsequent edition of this journal, we hope to promote a cross-disciplinary exchange of ideas with the thought that new ways of thinking from one field might ignite innovations in neighboring ones.

REFERENCES

Allen, K. R., & Walker, A. J. (1992). Attentive love: A feminist perspective on the caregiving of adult daughters. *Family Relations, 41*, 284–289.

Allen, R. I., & Petr, C. G. (1996). Toward developing standards and measurements for family-centered practice in family support programs. In G. H. S. Singer, L. E. Powers, & A. Olson (Eds.), *Redefining family support: Innovations in public-private partnerships* (pp. 57–86). Baltimore: Paul H. Brookes.

Americans with Disabilities Act of 1990 (ADA) (Pub.L. 101–336, 104 Stat.327, 42q U.S.C.§12101 et seq).

Arno, P., Levine, C., & Memmott, M. (1999). The economic value of informal caregiving. *Health Affairs, 18*(2), 182–188.

Bailey, D. B., Hebbeler, K., Scarborough, A., & Sangeeta, M. (2004). First experiences with early intervention: A national perspective. *Pediatrics, 113*(4), 887–896.

Biegel, D. E., Ishler, K., Katz, S., & Johnson, P. (2007). Predictors of burden in families of women with substance disorders or co-occurring substance and mental disorders. *Social Work Practice in the Addictions, 7*(1/2), 25–49.

Biegel, D. E., Robinson, E. M., & Kennedy, M. (2000). A review of empirical studies of interventions for families of persons with mental illness. In J. Morrisey (Ed.), *Research in Community Mental Health,* (Vol. 11, pp. 87–130). Greenwich, CT: JAI Press.

Biegel, D. E., Sales, E., & Schulz, R. (1991). Family caregiving in chronic illness: Alzheimer's disease, cancer, heart disease, mental illness, and stroke. *Family caregiver applications series 1*. Newbury Park, CA: Sage.

Blue-Banning, M., Summers, J. A., Frankland, C. H., Nelson, L. L., & Beegle, G. (2004). Dimensions of family and professional partnerships: Constructive guidelines for collaboration. *Exceptional Children, 20*(2), 167–184.

Bookman, A., & Harrington, M. (2007). Family caregivers: A shadow workforce in the geriatric health care system? *Journal of Health Politics, Policy, and Law, 32*(6), 1006–1041.

Boserup, E. (1970). *Women's role in economic development*. New York: St. Martins Press.

Braddock, D. L. (2002). Public financial support for disability at the dawn of the 21st century. *American Journal on Mental Retardation, 107*(6), 478–489.

Brown, R., Sherer, J., Wang, M., & Eacott, B. (in preparation). *A qualitative inquiry of family quality of life for individuals with intellectual disability in Australia.*

Carnevale, G. F., Anselmi, V., Busicio, K., & Millis, S. R. (2002). Changes in ratings of caregiver burden following a community-based behavior management program for persons with traumatic brain injury. *Journal of Head Trauma Rehabilitation, 17*(2), 83–95.

Caruth, A. K., Tate, U. S., Moffett, B. S., & Hill, K. (1997). Reciprocity, emotional well-being, and family functioning as determinants of family satisfaction in caregivers of elderly parents. *Nursing Research, 46*(2), 93–100.

Centers for Disease Control. (2008). *The prevalence of autism.* Retrieved September 16, 2008, from http://www.cdc.gov/ncbddd/autism/faq_prevalence.htm# whatisprevalence

Cooper, J. O., Heron, T. E., & Heward, W. L. (2007). *Applied behavior analysis* (2nd ed.). Upper Saddle River, NJ: Pearson.

Dixon, L., McFarlane, W. R., Lefley, H., Lucksted, A., Cohen, M., Falloon, I., et al. (2001). Evidence-based practices for services to families of people with psychiatric disabilities. *Psychiatric Services, 52*, 903–910.

Dunst, C. J., & Trivette, C. M. (in press). Using research evidence to inform and evaluate early childhood intervention practices. *Topics in Early Childhood Special Education.*

Dunst, C. J., Trivette, C. M., & Hamby, D. W. (2007). Meta-analysis of family-centered helpgiving practices research. *Mental Retardation and Developmental Disabilities Research Reviews, 13*(4), 370–378.

Edwards, A. B., Zarit, S. H., Stephens, M. A. P., & Townsend, A. (2002). Employed caregivers of cognitively impaired elderly: An examination of role strain and depressive symptoms. *Aging & Mental Health, 6*(1), 55–61.

Ethridge, B. L., & Singer, G. H. S. (2009). *Legislation mandating case management or other social work services to support family caregivers.* Manuscript in preparation.

Federal Interagency Forum on Aging-Related Statistics. (2008). *Older Americans 2008: Key indicators of well-being.* Washington, DC: U.S. Government Printing Office. Retrieved January 27, 2009 from http://www.agingstats.gov/agingstats dotnet/Main_Site/Data/2008_Documents/OA_2008.pdf

Fox, G. L., & Murry, V. M. (2000). Gender and families: Feminist perspectives and family research. *Journal of Marriage and the Family, 62*(4), 1160–1172.

Fujiura, G. T. (1998). Demography of family households. *American Journal on Mental Retardation, 103*(3), 225–35.

Gallagher-Thompson, D., & Coon, D. W. (2007). Evidence-based psychological treatments for distress in family caregivers of older adults. *Psychology & Aging, 22*(1), 37–51.

Gallimore, R., Weisner, T., Kaufman, S., & Bernheimer, L. (1989). The social construction of ecological niches: Family accommodation of developmentally delayed children. *American Journal of Mental Retardation, 94*, 216–230.

Greenberg, J. S., Greenley, J. R., & Benedict, P. (1994). Contributions of persons with serious mental illness to their families. *Hospital and Community Psychiatry, 45*(5), 475–480.

Hastings, R. P., & Taunt, H. M. (2002). Positive perceptions in families of children with developmental disabilities. *American Journal on Mental Retardation, 107*(2), 116–127.

Hooyman, N., & Gonyea, J. (1995). *Feminist perspectives on family care: Policies for gender justice*. Newbury Park, CA: Sage.

Ireys, H. T., Chernoff, R., DeVet, K. A., & Kim, Y. (2001). Maternal outcomes of a randomized controlled trial of community-based support program for families of children with chronic illnesses. *Archives of Pediatric Medicine, 155*, 771–777.

Jagger, C., Antony, A. J., Spiers, N. A., & Clarke, M. (2001). Patterns of onset of disability in activities of daily living with age. *Journal of the American Geriatrics Society, 49*(4), 404–409.

Kennedy, J., LaPlante, M., & Kaye, H. S. (1997). Need for assistance in the activities of daily living. *Disability Studies Abstracts, 18*, 2–5.

Keogh, B. K., Bernheimer, L. P., Gallimore, R., & Weisner, T. S. (1998). Child and family outcomes over time: A longitudinal perspective on developmental delays. In M. Lewis & C. Feiring (Eds.), *Families, risk and competence* (pp. 269–287). Mahwah, NJ: Erlbaum.

Kunkel, S. R., & Applebaum, R. A. (1999). *Estimating the prevalence of long-term disability for an aging society*. Washington, DC: U.S. Department of Health and Human Welfare, Office of Disability, Aging, and Long-term Care Policy. Retrieved September 17, 2008, from. http://aspe.hhs.gov/daltcp/reports/agsoces.pdf

Lefley, H. P. (in press). *Family psychoeducation for severe mental disorders*. New York: Oxford University Press.

Link, B. G., Mirotznik, J., & Cullen, F. T. (1991). The effectiveness of stigma coping orientations: Can negative consequences of mental illness labeling be avoided? *Journal of Health and Social Behavior, 32*, 302–320.

Losada, A., Izal, M., Perez-Rojo, G., & Montorio, I. (2007) Modification of dysfunctional thoughts about caregiving in dementia family caregivers: Description and outcomes of an intervention programme. *Aging & Mental Health, 11*(6), 616–625.

MacFarlane, W., Dixon, L., Lukens, E., & Lucksted, A. (2007). Family psychoeducation and schizophrenia: A review of the literature. *Journal of Marital and Family Therapy, 29*(2), 223–245.

McGraw, L. A., & Walker, A. J. (2004). Negotiating care: Ties between aging mothers and their caregiving daughters. *Journals of Gerontology: Social Sciences, 59B*, S324–S332.

McKeever, P. (1996). The family: Long-term care research and policy formation. *Nursing Inquiry, 3*, 200–206.

McWilliam, R. A., Lang, L., Vanderviere, P., Angel, R., Collins, L., & Underdown, G. (1995). Satisfaction and struggles: Family perceptions of early intervention services. *Journal of Early Intervention, 19*(1), 43–60.

MetLife Mature Market Institute and National Alliance for Caregiving. (2006). *The MetLife caregiving cost study: Productivity losses to U.S. business*. Bethesda, MD: National Alliance for Caregiving. Retrieved September 17, 2008, from http://www.caregiving.org/data/Caregiver%20Cost%20Study.pdf

National Alliance for Caregiving and AARP. (2004). *Caregiving in the U.S.* Retrieved September 16, 2008, from http://www.caregiving.org/data/04finalreport.pdf

National Alliance for the Mentally Ill (NAMI). (2006). *Grading the States: America's health care system for serious mental illness*. Arlington, VA: National Alliance on Mental Illness. Retrieved September 19, 2008, from http://www.nami.org/Content/NavigationMenu/Grading_the_States/Full_Report/GTS06_final.pdf

Neal, M. B., Chapman, N. J., Ingersoll-Dayton, B. I., & Emlen, A. C. (1993). *Balancing work and caregiving for children, adults, and elders*. Newbury Park, CA: Sage.

Newacheck, P. W., Kim, S. E., Blumberg, S. J., & Rising, J. P. (2008). Who is at risk for special health care needs: Findings from the National Survey of Children's Health. *Pediatrics, 122*(2), 347–359.

Novak, M., & Guest, C. (1989). Application of a multidimensional caregiver burden inventory. *The Gerontologist, 29*(6), 798–803.

Oakley, A. (1974). *The sociology of housework*. New York: Random House.

Older Americans Act, 42 USC Chapter 35 (2000).

Pandya, S. M. (2005). *Caregiving in the United States:* Fact sheet. Washington, DC: AARP Public Policy Institute. Retrieved September 15, 2008, from http://www.aarp.org/research/housingmobility/caregiving/fs111_caregiving.html

Powers, L., Singer, G. H. S., & Todis, B. (1996) Reflections on competence: Perspectives of successful adults. In L. E. Powers, G. H. S. Singer, & J. Sowers (Eds.), *On the road to autonomy* (pp. 69–92). Baltimore, MD: Paul H. Brookes.

Powers, L. E., Sowers, J., & Singer, G. H. S. (2006). A cross-disability analysis of person-directed, long-term services. *Journal of Disability Policy Studies, 17*(2), 66–76.

Romer, E. F., & Umbriet, J. (1998). The effects of family-centered service coordination: A social validity study. *Journal of Early Intervention, 21*(2), 95–110.

Ruddick, S. (1989). *Maternal thinking*. Boston: Beacon Press.

Schulz, R., & Beach, S. R. (1999). Caregiving as a risk factor for mortality: The caregiver health effects study. *Journal of the American Medical Association, 282*, 2215–2219.

Schulz, R. P., & Martire, L. M. (2004). Family caregiving of persons with dementia: Prevalence, health effects, and support. *American Journal of Geriatric Psychiatry, 12*(3), 240–249.

Seltzer, M. M., Greenberg, J. S., Floyd, F., Pettee, Y., & Hong, J. (2001). Life course impact of parenting a child with a disability. *American Journal on Mental Retardation, 106*(3), 265–286.

Seltzer, M. M., & Krauss, M. W. (2001). Quality of life on individuals with mental retardation/developmental disabilities who live with family. *Research Reviews in Mental Retardation and Developmental Disabilities, 7*, 105–114.

Singer, G. H. S. (2006). A meta-analysis of comparative studies of depression in mothers of children with developmental disabilities. *American Journal on Mental Retardation, 111*(3), 155–169.

Singer, G. H. S., Ethridge, B. L., & Aldana, S. I. (2007). Primary and secondary effects of parenting and stress management interventions for parents of children with developmental disabilities: A meta-analysis. *Mental Retardation and Developmental Disabilities Research Reviews, 13*(4), 357–369.

Singer, G. H. S., Goldberg-Hamblin, S., Peckham-Hardin, K. D., Barry, L., & Santarelli, G. E. (2002). Toward a synthesis of family support practices and positive behavior support. In J. Lucyshyn, G. Dunlap, & R. D. Albin (Eds.), *Families and positive behavior support: Addressing problem behavior in family contexts* (pp. 155–183). Baltimore, MD: Paul H. Brookes.

Singer, G. H. S., Powers, L. E., & Olson, A. (1996). *Redefining family support: Innovations in public-private partnerships*. Baltimore, MD: Paul H. Brookes.

Sorenson, S., Pinquart, M., & Duberstein, P. (2002). How effective are interventions with caregivers? An updated meta-analysis. *Gerontologist, 42*(3), 356–372.

Stock, L. Z., & Milan, M. A., (1993). Improving the dietary practices of elderly individuals: The power of prompting, feedback, and social reinforcement. *Journal of Applied Behavior Analysis, 26*(3), 379–387.

Townsend, A., Biegel, D. E., Ishler, K., Wieder, B., & Rini, A. (2006). Families of persons with substance and mental disorders: A conceptual framework and literature review. *Family Relations Journal, 55*, 473–486.

Turnbull, A. P., Turbiville, V., & Turnbull, H. R. (2000). *Evolution of family-professional partnership: collective empowerment as the model for the early twenty-first century*. In. J. P. Shonkoff & S. Miesels (Eds.), *The handbook of early childhood intervention* (2nd ed., pp. 630–650). Cambridge: Cambridge University Press.

U.S. Census Bureau. (2008). *Projected population of the United States, by age and sex: 2000–2050*. Retrieved September 16, 2008, from http://www.census.gov/statab/hist/HS-12.pdf

U.S. Department of Justice. (2008). *The Americans with Disability Act of 1990*. Retrieved September 17, 2008, from http://www.ada.gov/pubs/ada.htm#Anchor-Sec-11481

Velgouse, L., & Dize, V. (2000). A review of state initiatives in consumer-directed long-term care. *Generations, 24*(3), 28–34.

Walker, A. J., Pratt, C. C., & Eddy, L. (1995). Informal caregiving to aging family members: A critical review. *Family Relation, 44*(4), 402–411.

Wallander, J. L., Varni, J. W., Babani, L., Heatger, T. B., & Wilcox, K. T. (1989). Family resources as resistance factors for psychological maladjustment in chronically ill and handicapped children. *Journal of Pediatric Psychology, 14*(2), 157–173.

Witt, W. P., Riley, A. W., & Coiro, M. J. (2003). Childhood functional status, family stressors, and psychological adjustment among school-aged children with disabilities in the United States. *Archives of Pediatric Adolescent Medicine, 157*, 687–695.

Yell, M. (2006). *The law and special education*. Upper Saddle River, NJ: Pearson.

Capacity-Building Family-Systems Intervention Practices

CARL J. DUNST and CAROL M. TRIVETTE
Orelena Hawks Puckett Institute, Asheville, North Carolina

This article includes a description of a family-systems model for implementing early childhood and family support assessment and intervention practices. The model includes both conceptual and operational principles that link theory, research, and practice. Lessons learned from more than 20 years of research and practice have been used to revise and update the model, which now includes a major focus on family capacity building as a mediator of the benefits of intervention. Key components of the most recent version of the model are described, and findings from research syntheses showing the relationship between the different components of the family-systems model and parent, family, and child behavior and functioning are summarized. Future directions are described.

Contemporary interest in early childhood intervention with young children with disabilities and children at risk for poor developmental outcomes can be traced to a number of experimental studies conducted between 1940 and 1970 (for a review of these studies, see Dunst, 1996). The main goal of these, as well as subsequent intervention studies, was to lessen the effects of a disability or to prevent negative effects associated with poor environmental conditions. This was accomplished in the largest majority of studies by professionals intervening directly with young children or by professionals instructing parents on how to provide their children supplemental experiences deemed important for improving child functioning.

Most early childhood initiatives during the 1960s and 1970s, and even those in the 1980s, were based on an assumption that the children, their parents, or the environment were in some way deficit and that remedial measures were indicated (Lambie, Bond, & Weikart, 1975). It was also generally assumed that the interventions afforded the children would alleviate or reduce the consequences of the (presumed) deficits. The assumptions that constituted the foundations of these child-focused, deficit-based approaches to early childhood intervention were challenged by a number of experts (e.g., Foster, Berger, & McLean, 1981; Zigler & Berman, 1983), which became the basis of a new way of conceptualizing early childhood intervention. Bronfenbrenner (1975), for example, noted in his review of early childhood intervention programs, that the likelihood of these programs being successful is dependent, in part, on supporting parents who, in turn, would have the time and energy to promote their children's development.

More than 25 years ago, we began a process of transforming a deficit-based, child-focused early intervention program (Cornwell, Lane, & Swanton, 1975) into a strengths-based, family-focused early childhood intervention and family support program (see, e.g., Dunst, 1985; Trivette, Deal, & Dunst, 1986). The program began in 1972, and its practices were heavily influenced by deficit-based thinking at that time. Children were assessed to identify what they were not capable of doing, and professionals taught parents to use different techniques to promote children's behavior that were judged as lacking. In the early 1980s, as part of advances in family and systems theory (Bronfenbrenner, 1979), it became increasingly apparent that the family as well as the child needed to be the focus of intervention if the experiences afforded children and their families were likely to be optimally effective (Hobbs et al., 1984). The implications of the changes were a complete "rethinking" in how early childhood intervention and family support were conceptualized and implemented (Dunst, 1985).

The transformation we undertook was guided by key elements of *social-systems* (Bronfenbrenner, 1979), *empowerment* (Rappaport, 1981), *family strengths* (Stinnett & DeFrain, 1985), *social support* (Gottlieb, 1981), and *help-giving* (Brickman et al., 1982) theories. These different theories guided the conduct of research (e.g., Dunst, 1985; Dunst, Leet, & Trivette, 1988; Dunst & Trivette, 1988c; Dunst, Trivette, & Cross, 1986; Trivette & Dunst, 1987) as well as attempts to use key elements of the theories as part of interventions providing parents and other family members information, resources, advice, guidance, and other types of support to strengthen parenting and family functioning (e.g., Dunst, Cooper, & Bolick, 1987; Dunst & Trivette, 1987; Dunst & Trivette, 1988a; Dunst, Vance, & Cooper, 1986). One outcome of this research and practice was the publication of *Enabling and Empowering Families: Principles and Guidelines for Practice* (Dunst, Trivette, & Deal, 1988), which included methods and strategies for conceptualizing and implementing a family-systems approach to early childhood intervention and family support.

The purpose of this article is to describe a revised and updated version of the approach to early childhood intervention and family support described in *Enabling and Empowering Families*. The article is divided into three sections. The first includes an overview of the originally proposed model to provide a backdrop against which to understand the evolution and transformational features of the model. The second section includes a description of a revised and updated approach to supporting and strengthening families based on more than 20 years of lessons learned from both research and practice (e.g., Dunst, 2008; Dunst & Dempsey, 2007; Dunst, Hamby, & Brookfield, 2007; Trivette & Dunst, 2007a). The third section summarizes the results from meta-analyses of the relationships between the different components of the family-systems model and parent, family, and child behavior and functioning. The article concludes with thoughts about the future applicability of the model.

ENABLING AND EMPOWERING FAMILIES

Enabling and Empowering Families included sets of both conceptual and operational principles to structure an approach to working with families that used different kinds of enabling experiences and opportunities specifically intended to have empowering consequences and benefits (Rappaport, 1981). According to Brandtstädter (1980), conceptual principles "yield general rules for producing some desired effect, [whereas operative principles] supply decision aids for the effective implementation of [the] rules in the concrete action context" (p. 15). The conceptual principles, taken together, were intended to provide a framework for rethinking how and in what manner family-systems intervention practices were implemented. The operational principles constituted a set of assessment and intervention practices proposed to be easily used by professionals from different disciplines and backgrounds while working with families involved in early childhood intervention and family support programs.

Conceptual Principles

The eight conceptual principles constituting the foundations of *Enabling and Empowering Families* are the following:

1. Adoption of both a social-systems perspective of families and a family-systems definition of intervention. Accordingly, a family was viewed as a social unit embedded within other informal and formal social units and networks, where events in those units and networks reverberated and influenced the behavior of the family unit and individual family members (Bronfenbrenner, 1979). Intervention was defined as the "provision of support . . . from members of a family's informal and formal social

network that either directly or indirectly influenced child, parent, and family functioning" (Dunst, Trivette, & Deal, 1988, p. 5).

2. A focus on the family and not just a child as the unit of intervention. This principle was based on the fact that families who do not have the necessary supports and resources cannot adequately rear healthy, competent, and caring children (Hobbs et al., 1984). The provision of supports and resources to families was, in turn, expected to provide parents the time, energy, knowledge, and skills to provide their children development-enhancing learning opportunities (Bronfenbrenner, 1979).
3. Primary emphasis on family member empowerment as the goal of intervention. The premise of this principle is that a sense of control and mastery is an important mediator of behavior in many domains of functioning (Bandura, 1977). Empowerment was accomplished by creating opportunities for family members to acquire the knowledge and skills to better manage and negotiate daily living in ways positively affecting parent and family well-being and a sense of mastery and control (Rappaport, 1981).
4. Use of promotion rather than either treatment or prevention models for guiding intervention. This principle was based on the premise that the absence of problems was not the same as the presence of positive functioning (Bond, 1982). According to Carkhuff and Anthony (1979), helping is the act of promoting and supporting family functioning in a way that enhances the acquisition of competencies that permit a greater degree of control over subsequent life events and activities.
5. A focus on family and not professionally identified needs as the targets of intervention. This practice was derived from environmental press theory (Garbarino, 1982) that postulated the conditions under which people are motivated to address their needs. Accordingly, a practitioner did not assume a need for assistance until the family had set forth a need, where the request for assistance came from the family or individual family members (Pilisuk & Parks, 1986). The family-identified needs, in turn, were addressed by helping families use their strengths and capabilities to obtain the necessary resources and supports to meet needs.
6. Identify and build on family strengths as a way of supporting family functioning. This principle was based on the belief that all families have existing strengths and the capacity to become more competent (Rappaport, 1981), and that strengths-based interventions were likely to be more productive compared to attempts to prevent or correct weaknesses (Garbarino, 1982).
7. Using a family's informal social support network as a primary source of supports and resources for meeting family needs. This principle was based on a burgeoning body of evidence demonstrating the positive influences of support from family, friends, and neighbors on well-being and in other domains of functioning (e.g., Cohen & Syme, 1985; Sarason & Sarason,

1985). Therefore, to the extent possible and appropriate, informal supports were targeted as sources of information, guidance, assistance, and so on, because the "foresighted professional knows that it is the parent who truly bears the responsibility for the child, and the parent cannot be replaced by episodic professional services" (Hobbs, 1975, pp. 228–229).

8. Adoption of professional help-giving roles that place major emphasis on competency enhancement and the avoidance of dependencies. The premise of this principle was the contention that different kinds of helping beliefs and behaviors shaped and influenced interactions between professionals and families, and that certain help-giving practices were more likely to have competency enhancing effects (Brickman et al., 1982). As noted by Rappaport (1981), empowering help-giving practices require a breakdown in the typical relationships between professionals and families.

The delineation of these eight conceptual principles constituted an attempt to integrate the thinking of many noted experts and apply that thinking to the development of a family-systems approach to early childhood intervention and family support. The conceptual principles, in turn, were used to operationalize the principles in ways that mirrored or reflected the principles in action.

Operational Principles

The eight conceptual principles were used to develop an operational framework for guiding the conduct of family-systems assessment and intervention practices, as originally presented in *Enabling and Empowering Families* (see Figure 1). As stated in our book,

> "Family needs and aspirations, family strengths and capabilities (family functioning style), and social support and resources, are viewed as separate but interdependent parts of the assessment and intervention process. The help-giving behaviors used by professionals are the ways in which families are enabled and empowered to acquire and use competencies to procure supports and mobilize resources for meeting needs" (Dunst, Trivette, & Deal, 1988, p. 10).

The implementation of the assessment and intervention model was accomplished first by identifying family member needs and aspirations, second by identifying supports and resources for meeting needs, third by identifying existing and new strengths for obtaining resources and supports, and fourth by employing help-giving behaviors that strengthen family capacity to carry out actions intended to obtain supports and resources to meet self-identified needs.

Operational principles and goals of the assessment and intervention model are related (see Table 1). As noted in *Enabling and Empowering Families* (Dunst, Trivette, & Deal, 1988), the assessment and intervention

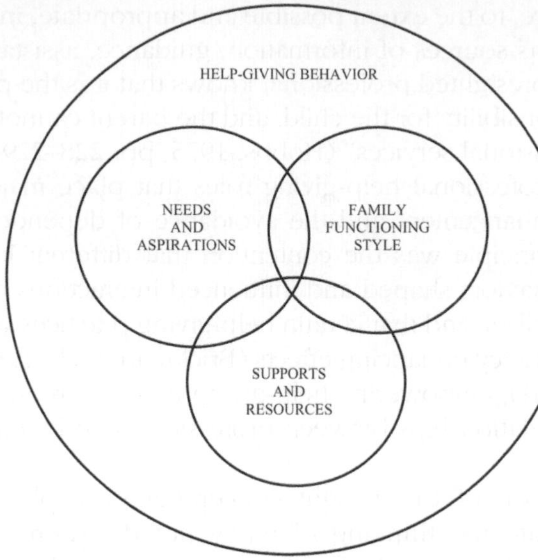

FIGURE 1 Family-systems assessment and intervention model constituting the focus of *Enabling and Empowering Families* (Dunst, Trivette, & Deal, 1988).

TABLE 1 Relationship Between the Four Operational Principles and Assessment and Intervention Goals of Each Family-Systems Model Component

Operational principles	Assessment and intervention goals
1. To promote positive child, parent, and family functioning, base interventions on family-identified needs, aspirations, personal projects, and priorities.	Identify family aspirations and priorities using needs-based assessment procedures and strategies to determine the things the family considers important enough to devote time and energy.
2. To insure the availability and adequacy of resources for meeting needs, place major emphasis on strengthening the family's personal social network as well as promoting utilization of untapped sources of information and assistance.	Identify family strengths and capabilities to (a) emphasize the things the family already does well and (b) determine the particular strengths that increase the likelihood of a family mobilizing resources to meet needs.
3. To enhance successful efforts toward meeting needs, use existing family functioning style (strengths and capabilities) as a basis for promoting the family's ability to obtain and mobilize resources.	"Map" the family's personal social network to identify both existing sources of support and resources and untapped but potential sources of aid and assistance.
4. To enhance a family's ability to become more self-sustaining with respect to meeting its needs, employ helping behaviors that promote the family's acquisition and use of competencies and skills necessary to mobilize and secure resources.	Function in a number of different help-giving roles to enable and empower the family to become more competent in mobilizing resources to meet its needs and achieve desired goals.

Source: Dunst et al. (1988, p. 53).

model is a "dynamic, fluid process" (p. 52) that involves different degrees of attention to each component of the model, depending on the emphasis of family member–help-giver exchanges. "The division of the assessment and intervention process into separate components was done primarily for heuristic purposes" (p. 52), because they are interdependent and require an integrated approach to assessment and intervention (Dunst, Trivette, & Deal, 1988).

Both interview and self-report assessment scales were used to identify family needs, family strengths, and sources of supports and resources for meeting needs. The purpose of the needs-assessment component of the model was to identify those family needs and aspirations that a family considered important enough to devote its time and energy. The purpose of the supports and resources component of the model was to identify the family, informal, and formal sources of supports and resources to meet needs. The purpose of the family strengths component of the model was to identify a family's capabilities that were used to obtain supports and resources to meet needs.

Twelve help-giving principles guided the ways in which professionals interacted with families while using the assessment and intervention practices (Dunst & Trivette, 1987). The help-giving principles were identified from an extensive review of the help-giving literature, with an explicit focus on those practices that were associated with empowerment-type outcomes and benefits (see especially Dunst & Trivette, 1988b; see Table 2). The help-giving behaviors, taken together, were viewed as the kinds of enabling

TABLE 2 Twelve Principles of Effective Help-giving

Help-giving is more likely to be effective when:

1. It is both positive and proactive and conveys a sincere sense of help giver warmth, caring, and encouragement.
2. It is offered in response to an indicated need for assistance.
3. Engages the help receiver in choice and decisions about the options best suited for obtaining desired supports and resources.
4. Is normative and typical of the help receivers' culture and values and is similar to how others would obtain assistance to meet similar needs.
5. It is congruent with how the help receiver views the appropriateness of the supports and resources for meeting needs.
6. The response–costs for seeking and accepting help do not outweigh the benefits.
7. Includes opportunities for reciprocating and the ability to limit indebtedness.
8. Bolsters the self-esteem of the help receiver by making resource and support procurement immediately successful.
9. Promotes, to the extent possible, the use of informal supports and resources for meeting needs.
10. Is provided in the context of help giver–help receiver collaboration.
11. It promotes the acquisition of effective behavior that decreases the need for the same type of help for the same kind of supports and resources.
12. It actively involves the help receiver in obtaining desired resource supports in ways bolstering his or her self-efficacy beliefs.

(in the good sense of the word) experiences and opportunities that would support and encourage parents' use of their strengths to obtain and procure desired supports and resources.

The assessment and intervention model was used in a variety of ways with families differing in needs, family structure, socioeconomic backgrounds, and other person and situational differences to evaluate its applicability and usefulness for supporting and strengthening family functioning. Lessons learned from the use of the family-systems model, as well as research investigating basic premises of the model, were in turn used to make changes and modifications in how the assessment and intervention model was conceptualized and implemented. The first set of changes are described in *Supporting and Strengthening Families: Methods, Strategies and Practices* (Dunst, Trivette, & Deal, 1994b).

PROMOTING AND ENHANCING FAMILY CAPACITY

The 20 years since the publication of *Enabling and Empowering Families* has provided us the opportunity to reflect on and refine its major tenets. Perhaps most surprising is the fact that nearly all the principles and practices have stood the test of time and still have value for guiding early childhood intervention and family support. Additional lessons learned from research and practice on the family-systems model have been used to further revise, refine, and update different elements of the model emphasizing those features that *matter most* in terms of having capacity-building characteristics and consequences. The emphasis on capacity building as both a process and benefit of family-systems assessment and intervention is based on research demonstrating that enabling experiences and opportunities positively influencing self-efficacy beliefs and other control appraisals mediate changes in many domains of life, including, but not limited to, parents' own judgments and capabilities to provide their children development-enhancing learning opportunities (Bandura, 1997; Skinner, 1995).

The updated version of the family-systems assessment and intervention model includes an operational definition of early childhood intervention and family support; a social-systems perspective of child, parent, and family behavior and functioning; a set of five different but compatible models that, taken together, constitute a capacity-building paradigm; and an operational framework for structuring the implementation of family-systems assessment and intervention practices. The key features of each of these elements are described next to illustrate advances in understanding of one particular approach to early childhood intervention and family support.

Definition of Early Childhood Intervention and Family Support

Early childhood intervention and family support are defined as the *provision or mobilization of supports and resources to families of young children from informal and formal social network members that either directly or indirectly influence and improve parent, family, and child behavior and functioning.* The experiences, opportunities, advice, guidance, and so forth afforded families by social network members are conceptualized broadly as different types of *interventions* contributing to improved functioning. The *sine qua non* outcome of the supports and resources afforded or procured by families includes any number of capacity-building and empowering consequences.

Our definition of intervention differs from most other definitions by its inclusion of informal supports as a focus of intervention and capacity building as a main consequence of the provision or mobilization of supports and resources. The inclusion of informal supports is based on research showing the manner in which these types of supports are related to improved parent and family functioning (for a review, see Dunst, Trivette, & Jodry, 1997). The focus on capacity building as an outcome of intervention is based on research demonstrating the manner in which different kinds of experiences and opportunities that have empowering characteristics and consequences, in turn, influence other dimensions of parent, family, and child behavior and functioning (Bandura, 1997; Dunst, Trivette, & Hamby, 2006, 2008; Skinner, 1995).

Our own research (e.g., Dunst, Trivette, Davis, & Cornwell, 1988; Dunst, Trivette, Starnes, Hamby, & Gordon, 1993), as well as that of others (e.g., Coyne & DeLongis, 1986; Galinsky & Schopler, 1994; Lincoln, 2000), has found that the manner in which support is provided, offered, or procured influences whether the support has positive, neutral or negative consequences. Affleck, Tennen, Rowe, Roscher, and Walker (1989) found that the provision of professional social support in response to an indicated need for assistance was associated with positive consequences, whereas the provision of social support in the absence of an indicated need for support had negative consequences. This is the basis, in part, for the identification of family concerns and priorities as the first step in our approach to family-systems assessment and intervention.

Systems Theory Framework

The provision or mobilization of supports and resources is accomplished in the context of a social systems framework, where a family is viewed as a social unit embedded within both informal and formal social support networks. According to Bronfenbrenner (1979), the behavior of a developing child, his or her parents, other family members, and the family unit as a whole are influenced by events occurring in settings beyond the family, which nonetheless directly and indirectly affect parent, family, and child behavior and functioning. Operationally, the supports and resources afforded families by informal and formal social support network members are defined as the experiences, opportunities, advice, guidance, material assistance, information, and so forth afforded or procured by family members that are intended to influence family member behaviors and functioning.

A basic premise of systems theory is that behavior is multiply determined and is a joint function of the characteristics of environmental experiences (supports and resources) and the person himself or herself (Bronfenbrenner, 1992). For example, research now indicates that the provision of help in response to an indicated need for support is likely to have positive consequences, whereas the provision of help in the absence of an indicated need for support is likely to have negative consequences (see especially Affleck, Tennen, Allen, & Gershman, 1986). Accordingly, the likelihood that an experience or opportunity afforded a person will have capacity-building influences is, in part, determined by an indicated need or desire for support and resources.

Capacity-Building Paradigm

Various attempts to operationalize and integrate different but compatible models of intervention led us to develop what we have come to call a *capacity-building paradigm* (see Table 3). These contrasting *worldviews* each have different implications for how interventions are conceptualized and implemented. The traditional worldview considers children and families as having deficits and weaknesses that need treatment by professionals to correct problems, whereas a capacity-building worldview considers children

TABLE 3 Defining Features of Contrasting Approaches for Conceptualizing and Implementing Early Childhood Intervention and Family Support Practices

Capacity-building paradigm	Traditional paradigm
Promotion models	*Treatment models*
Focus on enhancement and optimization of competence and positive functioning	Focus on remediation of a disorder, problem, or disease or its consequences
Empowerment models	*Expertise models*
Create opportunities for people to exercise existing capabilities as well as develop new competencies	Depend on professional expertise to solve problems for people
Strength-based models	*Deficit-based models*
Recognize the assets and talents of people and help people use these competencies to strengthen functioning	Focus on correcting peoples' weaknesses or problems
Resource-based models	*Service-based models*
Define practices in terms of a broad range of community opportunities and experiences	Define practices primarily in terms of professional services
Family-centered models	*Professionally centered models*
View professionals as agents of families who are responsive to family desires and concerns	View professionals as experts who determine the needs of people from their own as opposed to other peoples' perspectives

and families as having varied strengths and assets, where the focus of intervention is supporting and promoting competence and other positive aspects of family member functioning.

The models making up the capacity-building paradigm each include elements that place primary emphasis on the supports, resources, experiences, and opportunities afforded or provided children, parents, and families for strengthening existing, and promoting the acquisition of new competencies. Promotion models emphasize the enhancement of competence rather than the prevention or treatment of problems (Cowen, 1994; Dunst & Trivette, 2005; Dunst, Trivette, & Thompson, 1990). Empowerment models emphasize the kinds of experiences and opportunities that are contexts for competence expression (Dunst & Trivette, 1996; Zimmerman, 1990). Strengths-based models emphasize people's competence and how the use of different abilities and interests strengthen family member functioning (Dunst, 2008). Resource-based models emphasize a broad range of supports and resources (rather than services) as the experiences and opportunities for strengthening functioning (Dunst, Trivette, & Deal, 1994a; Raab, Davis, & Trepanier, 1993). Family-centered models emphasize the pivotal and central roles family members play in decisions about supports and resources best suited for improving parent, family, and child behavior and functioning (Dunst, 2002). Taken together, the five models provide a way of structuring the development and implementation of child and family intervention practices. The different models have proven useful for disentangling and unpacking what matters most in terms of those practices having desired consequences (e.g., Dunst, 2008; Dunst, Trivette, & Hamby, 2006; Dunst, Trivette, Hamby, & Bruder, 2006).

Family-Systems Intervention Model

The updated version of the four operational components of our family-systems assessment and intervention model are the same as those described in *Enabling and Empowering Families* but have been further refined based on research and practice (see Figure 2). The model is implemented by using capacity-building help-giving practices to identify family concerns and priorities, the supports and resources that can be used to address concerns and priorities, and the use of family member abilities and interests as the skills to obtain supports and resources.

The needs and aspirations component of the model has been changed to *family concerns and priorities* to reflect both families' dislike for the term need(y) and advances in our understanding of those life conditions that motivate people to alter or change their circumstances (Dunst & Deal, 1994). Concerns are defined as the perception or indication of a discrepancy between what is and what is desired. Priorities are defined as a condition that is judged highly important and deserving of attention. Both concerns and

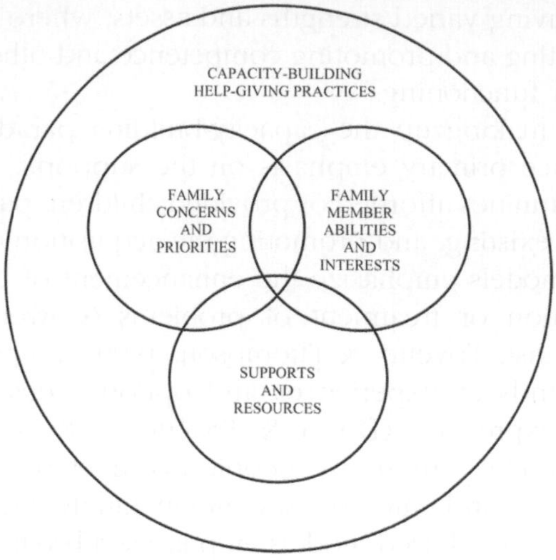

FIGURE 2 Major components of a capacity-building family-system assessment and intervention model.

priorities are viewed as determinants of how people spend time and energy seeking or obtaining resources and supports to achieve a desired goal or attain a particular end. While any number of terms have been used interchangeably to describe both concerns and priorities (Dunst & Deal, 1994), these particular terms cover the largest number of family situations that become the targets of intervention.

The *supports and resources* component of the model remains the same but has been redefined in terms of the kinds of assistance that constitute the information, instrumental assistance, experiences, opportunities, and so on, for addressing and responding to family concerns and priorities. The sources of support and resources still include both formal and informal social network members, with the caveat that family members are highly likely to seek out particular network members depending on which concerns and priorities are the focus of attention. The supports and resources deemed most appropriate are ones that actively involve family members in obtaining and procuring assistance rather than the noncontingent provision of help (see especially Dunst & Trivette, 1988b). It may seem expedient to provide or give families supports and resources, but doing so deprives them of opportunities to use existing skills or develop new competencies that can perpetuate a need for help (Skinner, 1978). To the extent that social network members "supply a needed resource but leads a person to see the production of that resource as contingent on what [others] do rather than his or her own behavior" (Brickman et al., 1983, p. 34), the support may have a negative or harmful consequence.

The family functioning style component has been changed to *family member abilities and interests* for two reasons. First, defining family strengths in terms of family qualities (Stinnett & DeFrain, 1985), family dynamic factors (Otto, 1963), and other qualitative family dimensions (Curran, 1983) has proven difficult to operationalize for many early childhood and family support practitioners. Second, our own research and practice (e.g., Dunst, 2008; Trivette & Dunst, 2007b), as well as that of others (e.g., Kretzmann & McKnight, 1993; Scales, Sesma, & Bolstrom, 2004), has found that defining family strengths in terms of specific abilities, interests, talents, and so on, makes the process of promoting family member identification and use of their strengths much more straightforward. We are still reminded of Stoneman's (1985) contention that "Every family has strengths and, if the emphasis [of intervention] is on supporting strengths rather than rectifying weaknesses, chances of making a difference in the lives of children are vastly increased" (p. 462).

The help-giving behavior component has been changed to *capacity-building help-giving practices* to reflect advances in our understanding of the particular kinds of help-giving practices that are most likely to have empowering characteristics and consequences. Research identifying the characteristics of effective help-giving practices has identified two clusters of help-giving that have capacity-building influences: *relational help-giving* and *participatory help-giving* (Trivette & Dunst, 2007a). Relational help-giving includes practices typically associated with good clinical practice (e.g., active listening, compassion, empathy, respect) and help-giver positive beliefs about family member strengths and capabilities. Listening to a family's concerns and asking for clarification or elaboration about what was said is an example of a relational help-giving practice. Participatory help-giving includes practices that are individualized, flexible, and responsive to family concerns and priorities, and which involve informed family choices and involvement in achieving desired goals and outcomes. Engaging a family member in a process of using information to make an informed decision about care for his or her child is an example of a participatory help-giving practice. Research syntheses of the relationships between both types of help-giving practices and parents' personal control appraisals and parent, family, and child behavior and functioning indicates that both types of helping practices are related to most outcomes. The results also showed that the relationship between relational and participatory help-giving and parent, family, and child behavior and functioning are mediated by personal control appraisals (Dunst, Trivette, & Hamby, 2007, 2008).

RESEARCH FOUNDATIONS

The extent to and manner in which the practices constituting the focus of each component of our family-systems assessment and intervention model are related to parent, family, and child behavior and functioning in a predicted manner has been the focus of a number of recently completed research syntheses (Dunst, Trivette, & Hamby, 2008; Dunst, Trivette, Hamby, & O'Herin, 2008; Hamby, Trivette, Dunst, & O'Herin, 2008; Trivette, Dunst, O'Herin, & Hamby, 2008). The analyses are briefly reported here and for the main effects between different measures of each of the four components of our family-systems model (help-giving, concerns, strengths, and supports) and the same or similar outcomes included in the different studies in the four meta-analyses.

Studies in the four syntheses were identified by searches of multiple electronic databases (Psychological Abstracts, ERIC, MEDLINE, Academic Search Elite, etc.), examination of seminal papers on each of the model components, and hand searches of key journals and all retrieved articles, chapters, and books. The average number of studies that were included in any one synthesis was 45 (range = 28–78). The average number of participants in the studies included in any one synthesis was 7,489 (range = 3012–10055).

The independent measures in the studies included different scales measuring capacity-building help-giving practices (e.g., Trivette & Dunst, 1994), family concerns (e.g., Dunst & Leet, 1985), family supports (e.g., Dunst, Jenkins, & Trivette, 1984), and family strengths (e.g., Deal, Trivette, & Dunst, 1988). All the scales used to measure the independent variables, except those in the Dunst, Trivette, and Hamby (2008) meta-analyses of family-centered help-giving practices, were instruments we developed or have used in studies we and our colleagues have conducted.

The help-giving practices scales included measures of help-giver active listening and empathy, help-receiver choice and decision making, help giver–help receiver collaboration, and help-receiver active involvement in obtaining desired supports and resources. The family concerns scales included measures of an indicated need for basic resources (e.g., food and shelter), employment and financial resources, health and dental care, child care, time for self and family, and dependable transportation. The family strengths scales included measures of family commitment, problem-solving strategies, patterns of interaction, coping strategies, and family values. The social support scales included measures of support from spouse or partner, family members and other kin, friends and neighbors, church members and coworkers, early childhood programs and practitioners, and parent and social groups.

The dependent measures in the studies were grouped into five categories: personal control and self-efficacy, parent well-being, parenting, family functioning, and child behavior. The personal control and self-efficacy belief measures included scales measuring control over general life events (e.g., Boyd & Dunst, 1996; Nowicki & Duke, 1974). The parent well-being measures included scales assessing stress, depression, and other adverse psychological states (e.g., Abidin, 1990; Radloff, 1977). The parenting scales measured different aspects of parent competence and confidence (e.g., Dunst & Masiello, 2002; Guidubaldi & Cleminshaw, 1994). The family functioning scales included measures of family cohesion, integration, and well-being (e.g., Hampson & Hulgus, 1986; McCubbin & Comeau, 1987). The child behavior scales measured different aspects of positive and negative child functioning (e.g., Achenbach, 1993; Conners, 1997). The particular dependent measures in the analyses presented here are ones that were included in at least three of the four meta-analyses so that comparisons of the relationships between the family-system model component measures and the same or similar outcomes could be made.

The correlations between the independent and dependent measures were used as the sizes of effects for the relationships between the family-systems components and the dependent measures (Rosenthal, 1994). The direction of the correlations between measures were coded so that a positive correlation between the independent and dependent measures represented more positive and less negative behavior functioning. Procedures described by Shadish and Haddock (1994) were used to combine effect sizes, giving more weight to studies with larger sample sizes. The average weighted effect sizes were used as the best estimate of the strength of the relationship between measures. Data interpretation was aided by the 95% confidence intervals of the average weighted effect sizes. An interval not including zero indicates that the average size of effect is statistically different from zero at the .05 level (Hedges, 1994).

The average weighted effect sizes between the component measures and the outcomes were all significantly different from zero as evidenced by no confidence intervals including zero (see Figure 3). Stated differently, variations in the measures of each family-systems component were related to variations in the outcomes in ways that were expected. The more the study participants experienced capacity-building help-giving practices, the better the outcomes; the fewer concerns the study participants reported, the better the outcomes; the more family strengths the study participants reported, the better the outcomes; and the more social support that was available to the study participants and their families, the better the outcomes. The patterns of relationships and sizes of effects, however, were not the same as evidenced by the unevenness in the strength of the relationships between the independent and dependent measures, which are briefly described next.

The size of the effect between help-giving practices and self-efficacy beliefs was more than twice as large as the relationships between either family concerns or social supports and this same outcome. The fact that help-giving practices were more strongly related to self-efficacy beliefs was not unexpected, inasmuch as this has consistently been found as part of this line of research (see especially Dunst, Trivette, & Hamby, 2006; 2007; Dunst, Trivette, & Hamby, 2008).

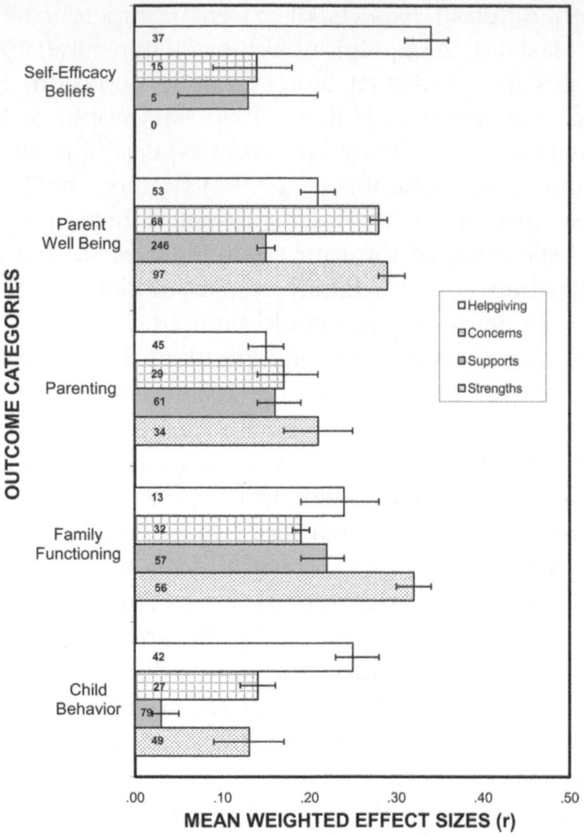

FIGURE 3 Average weighted effect sizes and 95% confidence intervals for the relationships between the four family-systems model components (independent variables) and five categories of parent, family, and child outcomes (dependent measures). (*Note*: The numbers on the bars are the number of effect sizes included in the analyses).

Family strengths were more strongly related to family functioning compared to the other family-systems component measures, whereas help-giving practices were more strongly related to child behavior and functioning compared to the other family-systems components measures. Both family concerns and family strengths were more strongly related to parent well-being compared to the relationships between either help-giving practices or social supports and this same outcome. In contrast, all four family-systems component measures were more similarly related to the parenting outcome measures.

The fact that there were differential relationships between measures was not unexpected. This has been the rule rather than the exception in nearly every kind of analysis we have performed on measures of the family-systems model components. The differential relationships between measures indicate that the four family-systems practices components each exert different influences on parent, family, and child behavior and functioning. Despite the differential influences of each type of practice, the findings, taken together, show that measures of each component of the family-system model are related to parent, family, and child behavior and functioning in a manner consistent with predictions from the conceptual frameworks guiding both our research and practice (e.g., Dunst, 1997; Dunst et al., 1990; Trivette, Dunst, & Deal, 1997; Trivette, Dunst, & Hamby, 1996).

CONCLUSIONS

The family-systems model as well as specific components of the model have been evaluated as part of many different child, parent, and family intervention studies (e.g., Dunst, 2001, 2008; Dunst et al., 2001; Dunst, Masiello, & Murillo, 2008; Dunst, Raab, et al., 2007; Dunst & Trivette, 2001; Dunst, Trivette, Gordon, & Pletcher, 1989). The main focus of these and other studies was the identification of the conditions under which needs-based, social support, strengths-based, and capacity-building help-giving interventions and practices were likely to be most effective. A lesson learned from these intervention studies was the fact that the more straightforward the interventions, the higher the probability that the interventions would be implemented as planned and intended, and have expected benefits. This was likely the case because "there is evidence that it is easier to achieve high fidelity of simple [rather] than complex interventions . . . because there are fewer 'response barriers' when the model is simple" (Carroll et al., 2007).

A few examples should help elucidate the contention that "less is more" when using family-systems assessment and intervention practices. In an intervention study of teenage mothers involved in a parenting support program, the participants were enrolled in a work-study program (infant and preschool classrooms) where they had the opportunity to observe and work with teachers who interacted with children in development-enhancing manners (Dunst, Vance, et al., 1986). Over the course of just 20 weeks, the teenage mothers increasingly used the same kinds of interactional styles observed in the classrooms with their own children. In an intervention study of parents from extremely low socioeconomic backgrounds, the parents' strengths (abilities and interests) were used as sources of young children's learning opportunities (Dunst, 2008). Results showed increases in the learning opportunities afforded the children, and both child and parent positive behavioral consequences. Similar kinds of straightforward interventions have also been found to also have positive effects (e.g., Bakermans-Kranenburg, van IJzendoorn, & Juffer, 2003).

Following the publication of *Enabling and Empowering Families,* and in the intervening 20 years, we became aware of numerous attempts by others to use the principles and practices we articulated in our book with families from many different cultural and ethnic backgrounds, with families in different countries, with children and families with varying life circumstances and conditions, and by practitioners in many different kinds of early childhood intervention, family support, health, and human services programs (e.g., Coutinho, 2004; DePanfilis, 1998; Hossain, 2001; Kalyanpur & Rao, 1991; McCarthy et al., 2002; Mitchell & Sloper, 2002; Sheridan, Warnes, Cowan, Schemm, & Clarke, 2004). At the time *Enabling and Empowering Families* was written, we strived to develop a model and a set of principles and practices that were flexible enough to be used in different settings and contexts with families having diverse backgrounds and life circumstances. The flexibility we had hoped to achieve is reflected, at least in part, by the broad-based use of the family-systems assessment and intervention model.

One focus of our current research on family-systems intervention is further evaluations of the relationships between the model components and the extent to which different elements of each component have either or both direct and indirect effects on parent, family, and child behavior and functioning. This is being accomplished by both structural equation modeling of data from studies we have conducted (see e.g., Dunst, 1999; Dunst, Hamby et al., 2007; Trivette et al., 1996) and meta-analytic structural equation modeling (Cheung & Chan, 2005; Shadish, 1996) of studies conducted by ourselves and others examining the relationships between two or more components of our model and child, parent, or family outcomes. The goal is a better understanding of how the family-systems components are related and the conditions under which optimal benefits are realized. The expected outcome of this next generation of research is the isolation of those component characteristics that matter most in terms of having predicted effects and both the disentangling and unpacking of how the different components are related to one another, and, in turn, influence parent, family, and child behavior and functioning. Findings from these efforts will be used to completely revise *Enabling and Empowering Families* with a focus on the key ingredient practices and how they can be implemented to best support and strengthen child, parent, and family functioning.

REFERENCES

Abidin, R. (1990). *Parenting stress index: Manual* (3rd ed.). Charlottesville, VA: Pediatric Psychology Press.

Achenbach, T. M. (1993). *Manual for the child behavior checklist.* Burlington, VT: Author.

Affleck, G., Tennen, H., Allen, D. A., & Gershman, K. (1986). Perceived social support and maternal adaptation during the transition from hospital to home care of high-risk infants. *Infant Mental Health Journal, 7*, 6–18.

Affleck, G., Tennen, H., Rowe, J., Roscher, B., & Walker, L. (1989). Effects of formal support on mothers' adaptation to the hospital-to-home transition of high-risk infants: The benefits and costs of helping. *Child Development, 60*, 488–501.

Bakermans-Kranenburg, M. J., van IJzendoorn, M. H., & Juffer, F. (2003). Less is more: Meta-analyses of sensitivity and attachment interventions in early childhood. *Psychological Bulletin, 129*, 195–215.

Bandura, A. (1977). Self-efficacy: Toward a unifying theory of behavioral change. *Psychological Review, 84*, 191–215.

Bandura, A. (1997). *Self-efficacy: The exercise of control*. New York: Freeman.

Bond, L. A. (1982). From prevention to promotion: Optimizing infant development. In G. W. Albee & J. M. Joffe (Eds.), *Primary prevention of psychopathology: Vol. VI. Facilitating infant and early childhood development* (pp. 5–39). Hanover, NH: University Press of New England.

Boyd, K., & Dunst, C. J. (1996). *Personal assessment of control scale*. Asheville, NC: Winterberry Press.

Brandtstädter, J. (1980). Relationships between life-span developmental theory, research, and intervention: A revision of some stereotypes. In R. R. Turner & H. W. Reese (Eds.), *Life-span developmental psychology* (pp. 3–28). New York: Academic.

Brickman, P., Kidder, L. H., Coates, D., Rabinowitz, V., Cohn, E., & Karuza, J. (1983). The dilemmas of helping: Making aid fair and effective. In J. D. Fisher, A. Nadler, & B. M. DePaulo (Eds.), *New directions in helping: Vol. 1. Recipient reactions to aid* (pp. 17–49). New York: Academic Press.

Brickman, P., Rabinowitz, V. C., Karuza, J., Jr., Coates, D., Cohn, E., & Kidder, L. (1982). Models of helping and coping. *American Psychologist, 37*, 368–384.

Bronfenbrenner, U. 1975. Is early intervention effective? In B. Z. Friedlander, G. M. Sterritt, & G. E. Kirk (Eds.), *Exceptional infant: Vol. 3. Assessment and intervention* (pp. 449–475). New York: Brunner/Mazel.

Bronfenbrenner, U. (1979). *The ecology of human development: Experiments by nature and design*. Cambridge, MA: Harvard University Press.

Bronfenbrenner, U. (1992). Ecological systems theory. In R. Vasta (Ed.), *Six theories of child development: Revised formulations and current issues* (pp. 187–248). Philadelphia: Jessica Kingsley.

Carkhuff, R. R., & Anthony, W. A. (1979). *The skills of helping*. Amherst, MA: Human Resource Development Press.

Carroll, C., Patterson, M., Wood, S., Booth, A., Rick, J., & Balain, S. (2007). A conceptual framework for implementation fidelity. *Implementation Science, 2*, 40. Retrieved February 19, 2008, from http://www.implementationscience.com/content/pdf/1748-5908-2-40.pdf

Cheung, M. W., & Chan, W. (2005). Meta-analytic structural equation modeling: A two-stage approach. *Psychological Methods, 10*(1), 40–64.

Cohen, S., & Syme, S. L. (Eds.). (1985). *Social support and health*. Orlando, FL: Academic Press.

Conners, C. K. (1997). *Conners' parent rating scale*. North Tonawanda, NY: Multi-Health Systems.

Cornwell, S., Lane, A., & Swanton, C. (1975). A home-centered regional program for developmentally impaired infants and toddlers. *North Carolina Journal of Mental Health, 7*, 56–65.

Coutinho, M. T. B. (2004). Apoio à família e formação parental. *Analise Psicologica, 22*, 55–64.

Cowen, E. L. (1994). The enhancement of psychological wellness: Challenges and opportunities. *American Journal of Community Psychology, 22*, 149–179.

Coyne, J. C., & DeLongis, A. (1986). Going beyond social support: The role of social relationships in adaptation. *Journal of Consulting and Clinical Psychology, 54*, 454–460.

Curran, D. (1983). *Traits of a healthy family: Fifteen traits commonly found in healthy families by those who work with them*. Minneapolis, MN: Winston Press.

Deal, A. G., Trivette, C. M., & Dunst, C. J. (1988). *Family Functioning Style Scale: An instrument for measuring strengths and resources*. Asheville, NC: Winterberry Press.

DePanfilis, D. 1998, November. *Structured decision making and risk assessment: Assessing neglect*. Presentation made at the 12th National Conference on Child Abuse and Neglect, Cincinnati, OH.

Dunst, C. J. (1985). Rethinking early intervention. *Analysis and Intervention in Developmental Disabilities, 5*, 165–201.

Dunst, C. J. (1996). Early intervention in the USA: Programs, models, and practices. In M. Brambring, H. Rauh, & A. Beelmann (Eds.), *Early childhood intervention: Theory, evaluation, and practice* (pp. 11–52). Berlin, Germany: de Gruyter.

Dunst, C. J. (1997). Conceptual and empirical foundations of family-centered practice. In R. Illback, C. Cobb, & H. Joseph, Jr. (Eds.), *Integrated services for children and families: Opportunities for psychological practice* (pp. 75–91). Washington, DC: American Psychological Association.

Dunst, C. J. (1999). Placing parent education in conceptual and empirical context. *Topics in Early Childhood Special Education, 19*, 141–147.

Dunst, C. J. (2001). Participation of young children with disabilities in community learning activities. In M. J. Guralnick (Ed.), *Early childhood inclusion: Focus on change* (pp. 307–333). Baltimore: Brookes.

Dunst, C. J. (2002). Family-centered practices: Birth through high school. *Journal of Special Education, 36*, 139–147.

Dunst, C. J. (2008). *Parent and community assets as sources of young children's learning opportunities* (Rev. and expanded ed.). Asheville, NC: Winterberry Press.

Dunst, C. J., Bruder, M. B., Trivette, C. M., Hamby, D., Raab, M., & McLean, M. (2001). Characteristics and consequences of everyday natural learning opportunities. *Topics in Early Childhood Special Education, 21*, 68–92.

Dunst, C. J., Cooper, C. S., & Bolick, F. A. (1987). Supporting families of handicapped children. In J. Garbarino, P. Brookhouser, & K. Authier (Eds.), *Special children—special risks: The maltreatment of children with disabilities* (pp. 17–46). New York: de Gruyter.

Dunst, C. J., & Deal, A. G. (1994). Needs-based family-centered intervention practices. In C. J. Dunst, C. M. Trivette, & A. G. Deal (Eds.), *Supporting and strengthening families: Methods, strategies and practices* (pp. 90–104). Cambridge, MA: Brookline Books.

Dunst, C. J., & Dempsey, I. (2007). Family-professional partnerships and parenting competence, confidence, and enjoyment. *International Journal of Disability, Development, and Education, 54*, 305–318.

Dunst, C. J., Hamby, D. W., & Brookfield, J. (2007). Modeling the effects of early childhood intervention variables on parent and family well-being. *Journal of Applied Quantitative Methods, 2*, 268–288.

Dunst, C. J., Jenkins, V., & Trivette, C. (1984). *Family Support Scale*. Asheville, NC: Winterberry Press.

Dunst, C. J., & Leet, H. E. (1985). *Family Resource Scale: Reliability and validity*. Asheville, NC: Winterberry Press.

Dunst, C. J., Leet, H. E., & Trivette, C. M. (1988). Family resources, personal well-being, and early intervention. *Journal of Special Education, 22*, 108–116.

Dunst, C. J., & Masiello, T. L. (2002). *Everyday parenting scale*. Asheville, NC: Winterberry Press.

Dunst, C. J., Masiello, T. L., & Murillo, M. 2008. *Parental personal assets: Contexts for children's everyday learning*. Manuscript in preparation.

Dunst, C. J., Raab, M., Trivette, C. M., Wilson, L. L., Hamby, D. W., Parkey, C., Gatens, M., & French, J. (2007). Characteristics of operant learning games associated with optimal child and adult social-emotional consequences [Electronic version]. *International Journal of Special Education, 22*(3), 13–24.

Dunst, C. J., & Trivette, C. M. (1987). Enabling and empowering families: Conceptual and intervention issues. *School Psychology Review, 16*, 443–456.

Dunst, C. J., & Trivette, C. M. (1988a). A family systems model of early intervention with handicapped and developmentally at-risk children. In D. R. Powell (Ed.), *Parent education as early childhood intervention: Emerging directions in theory, research, and practice* (pp. 131–179). Norwood, NJ: Ablex.

Dunst, C. J., & Trivette, C. M. (1988b). Helping, helplessness, and harm. In J. C. Witt, S. N. Elliott, & F. M. Gresham (Eds.), *Handbook of behavior therapy in education* (pp. 343–376). New York: Plenum Press.

Dunst, C. J., & Trivette, C. M. (1988c). Toward experimental evaluation of the family, infant and preschool program. In H. B. Weiss & F. H. Jacobs (Eds.), *Evaluating family programs* (pp. 315–346). New York: de Gruyter.

Dunst, C. J., & Trivette, C. M. 1996. Empowerment, effective help-giving practices and family-centered care. *Pediatric Nursing, 22*, 334–337, 343.

Dunst, C. J., & Trivette, C. M. (2001). *Benefits associated with family resource center practices*. Asheville, NC: Winterberry Press.

Dunst, C. J., & Trivette, C. M. 2005. Family resource programs, promotion models, and enhancement outcomes. *Practical Evaluation Reports, 1*(1), 1–5. Retrieved May 23, 2006, from http://www.practicalevaluation.org/reports/cpereport_vol1_no1.pdf

Dunst, C. J., Trivette, C. M., & Cross, A. H. (1986). Mediating influences of social support: Personal, family, and child outcomes. *American Journal of Mental Deficiency, 90*, 403–417.

Dunst, C. J., Trivette, C. M., Davis, M., & Cornwell, J. (1988). Enabling and empowering families of children with health impairments. *Children's Health Care, 17*, 71–81.

Dunst, C. J., Trivette, C. M., & Deal, A. (1988). *Enabling and empowering families: Principles and guidelines for practice*. Cambridge, MA: Brookline Books.

Dunst, C. J., Trivette, C. M., & Deal, A. G. (1994a). Resource-based family-centered intervention practices. In C. J. Dunst, C. M. Trivette, & A. G. Deal (Eds.), *Supporting and strengthening families: Methods, strategies and practices* (pp. 140–151). Cambridge, MA: Brookline Books.

Dunst, C. J., Trivette, C. M., & Deal, A. G. (Eds.). (1994b). *Supporting and strengthening families: Methods, strategies and practices*. Cambridge, MA: Brookline Books.

Dunst, C. J., Trivette, C. M., Gordon, N. J., & Pletcher, L. L. (1989). Building and mobilizing informal family support networks. In G. H. Singer & L. Irvin (Eds.), *Support for caregiving families: Enabling positive adaptation to disability* (pp. 121–141). Baltimore, MD: Brookes.

Dunst, C. J., Trivette, C. M., & Hamby, D. W. (2006). *Family support program quality and parent, family and child benefits* (Winterberry Monograph Series). Asheville, NC: Winterberry Press.

Dunst, C. J., Trivette, C. M., & Hamby, D. W. (2007). Meta-analysis of family-centered help-giving practices research. *Mental Retardation and Developmental Disabilities Research Reviews*, *13*, 370–378.

Dunst, C. J., Trivette, C. M., & Hamby, D. W. (2008). *Research synthesis and meta-analysis of studies of family-centered practices* (Winterberry Monograph Series). Asheville, NC: Winterberry Press.

Dunst, C. J., Trivette, C. M., Hamby, D. W., & Bruder, M. B. (2006). Influences of contrasting natural learning environment experiences on child, parent, and family well-being. *Journal of Developmental and Physical Disabilities*, *18*, 235–250.

Dunst, C. J., Trivette, C. M., Hamby, D. W., & O'Herin, C. E. (2008). *Research synthesis of the relationship between family needs and parent, family and child outcomes* (Winterberry Research Sytheses). Asheville, NC: Winterberry Press. (in preparation).

Dunst, C. J., Trivette, C. M., & Jodry, W. (1997). Influences of social support on children with disabilities and their families. In M. Guralnick (Ed.), *The effectiveness of early intervention* (pp. 499–522). Baltimore, MD: Brookes.

Dunst, C. J., Trivette, C. M., Starnes, A. L., Hamby, D. W., & Gordon, N. J. (1993). *Building and evaluating family support initiatives: A national study of programs for persons with developmental disabilities*. Baltimore: Brookes.

Dunst, C. J., Trivette, C. M., & Thompson, R. B. (1990). Supporting and strengthening family functioning: Toward a congruence between principles and practice. *Prevention in Human Services*, *9*(1), 19–43.

Dunst, C. J., Vance, S. D., & Cooper, C. S. (1986). A social systems perspective of adolescent pregnancy: Determinants of parent and parent-child behavior. *Infant Mental Health Journal*, *7*, 34–48.

Foster, M., Berger, M., & McLean, M. (1981). Rethinking a good idea: A reassessment of parent involvement. *Topics in Early Childhood Special Education*, *1*(3), 55–65.

Galinsky, M. J., & Schopler, J. H. (1994). Negative experiences in support groups. *Social Work in Health Care*, *20*, 77–95.

Garbarino, J. (1982). *Children and families in the social environment*. New York: Aldine.

Gottlieb, B. H. (1981). *Social networks and social support*. Beverly Hills, CA: Sage.

Guidubaldi, J., & Cleminshaw, H. K. (1994). *Parenting satisfaction scale*. San Antonio, TX: Psychological Corporation.

Hamby, D. W., Trivette, C. M., Dunst, C. J., & O'Herin, C. E. (2008). *Relationship between social support and parent, family and child benefits: A meta-analysis* (Winterberry Research Syntheses). Asheville, NC: Winterberry Press. (in preparation).

Hampson, R. B., & Hulgus, Y. F. (1986). *Psychometric evaluation of the self-report family inventory*. Dallas, TX: Southwest Family Institute.

Hedges, L. V. (1994). Fixed effects models. In H. Cooper & L. V. Hedges (Eds.), *The handbook of research synthesis* (pp. 285–299). New York: Russell Sage Foundation.

Hobbs, N. (1975). *The futures of children: Categories, labels, and their consequences*. San Francisco, CA: Jossey-Bass.

Hobbs, N., Dokecki, P. R., Hoover-Dempsey, K. V., Moroney, R. M., Shayne, M. W., & Weeks, K. H. (1984). *Strengthening families*. San Francisco, CA: Jossey-Bass.

Hossain, Z. (2001). Division of household labor and family functioning in off-reservation Navajo Indian families. *Family Relations, 50*, 255–261.

Kalyanpur, M., & Rao, S. S. (1991). Empowering low-income Black families of handicapped children. *American Journal of Orthopsychiatry, 61*, 523–532.

Kretzmann, J. P., & McKnight, J. (1993). *Building communities from the inside out: A path toward finding and mobilizing a community's assets*. Chicago, IL: ACTA.

Lambie, D. Z., Bond, J. T., & Weikart, D. P. (1975). Framework for infant education. In B. Z. Friedlander, G. M. Steritt, & G. E. Kirk (Eds.), *Exceptional infant: Volume 3* (pp. 263–284). New York: Brunner/Mazel.

Lincoln, K. D. (2000). Social support, negative social interactions, and psychological well-being. *Social Service Review, 74*, 231–252.

McCarthy, M. J., Herbert, R., Brimacombe, M., Hansen, J., Wong, D. L., & Zelman, M. (2002). Empowering parents through asthma education. *Pediatric Nursing, 28*, 465–474.

McCubbin, H. I., & Comeau, J. K. (1987). FIRM: Family inventory of resources for management. In H. I. McCubbin & A. I. Thompson (Eds.), *Family assessment inventories for research and practice* (pp. 158–160). Madison: University of Wisconsin.

Mitchell, W., & Sloper, P. (2002). Information that informs rather than alienates families with disabled children: Developing a model of good practice. *Health and Social Care in the Community, 10*, 74–81.

Nowicki, S., & Duke, M. P. (1974). A locus of control scale for noncollege as well as college adults. *Journal of Personality Assessment, 38*, 136–137.

Otto, H. A. (1963). Criteria for assessing family strengths. *Family Process, 2*, 329–334.

Pilisuk, M., & Parks, S. H. (1986). *The healing web: Social networks and human survival*. Hanover, NH: University Press of New England.

Raab, M. M., Davis, M. S., & Trepanier, A. M. (1993). Resources vs. services: Changing the focus of intervention with infants and toddlers with special needs. *Infants and Young Children, 5*(3), 1–11.

Radloff, L. S. (1977). *Center for Epidemiological Studies depression scale (short form)*. Unpublished scale, National Institute of Mental Health.

Rappaport, J. (1981). In praise of paradox: A social policy of empowerment over prevention. *American Journal of Community Psychology, 9*, 1–25.

Rosenthal, R. (1994). Parametric measures of effect size. In H. Cooper & L. V. Hedges (Eds.), *The handbook of research synthesis* (pp. 231–244). New York: Russell Sage Foundation.

Sarason, I. G., & Sarason, B. R. (Eds.). (1985). *Social support: Theory, research and applications*. Dordrecht, The Netherlands: Martinus Nijhoff.

Scales, P. C., Sesma, A., Jr., & Bolstrom, B. (2004). *Coming into their own: How developmental assets promote positive growth in middle childhood*. Minneapolis, MN: Search Institute.

Shadish, W. R. (1996). Meta-analysis and the exploration of causal mediating processes: A primer of examples, methods, and issues. *Psychological Methods, 1*, 47–65.

Shadish, W. R., & Haddock, C. K. (1994). Combining estimates of effect size. In H. Cooper & L. V. Hedges (Eds.), *The handbook of research synthesis* (pp. 261–281). New York: Russell Sage Foundation.

Sheridan, S. M., Warnes, E. D., Cowan, R. J., Schemm, A. V., & Clarke, B. L. (2004). Family-centered positive psychology: Focusing on strengths to build student success. *Psychology in the Schools, 41*, 7–17.

Skinner, B. F. (1978). The ethics of helping people. In L. Wispé (Ed.), *Altruism, sympathy, and helping: Psychological and sociological principles* (pp. 249–262). New York: Academic Press.

Skinner, E. A. (1995). *Perceived control, motivation, and coping*. Thousand Oaks, CA: Sage.

Stinnett, N., & DeFrain, J. (1985). *Secrets of strong families*. Boston: Little, Brown.

Stoneman, Z. (1985). Family involvement in early childhood special education programs. In N. Fallen & W. Umansky (Eds.), *Young children with special needs* (2nd ed., pp. 442–469). Columbus, OH: Charles Merrill.

Trivette, C. M., Deal, A., & Dunst, C. J. (1986). Family needs, sources of support, and professional roles: Critical elements of family systems assessment and intervention. *Diagnostique, 11*, 246–267.

Trivette, C. M., & Dunst, C. J. (1987). Proactive influences of social support in families of handicapped children. In H. G. Lingren, L. Kimmons, P. Lee, G. Rowe, L. Rottmann, L. Schwab, & R. Williams (Eds.), *Family strengths: Vol. 8–9. Pathways to well-being* (pp. 391–405). Lincoln: University of Nebraska, Center for Family Strengths.

Trivette, C. M., & Dunst, C. J. (1994). *Helpgiving practices scale*. Asheville, NC: Winterberry Press.

Trivette, C. M., & Dunst, C. J. (2007a). *Capacity-building family-centered help-giving practices* (Winterberry Research Reports Vol. 1, No. 1). Asheville, NC: Winterberry Press.

Trivette, C. M., & Dunst, C. J. (2007b, May). *Family strengths in different cultures*. Presentation made at Building Family Strengths: Research and Services in Support of Children and their Families Conference, Portland, OR.

Trivette, C. M., Dunst, C. J., & Deal, A. G. (1997). Resource-based approach to early intervention. In S. K. Thurman, J. R. Cornwell, & S. R. Gottwald (Eds.), *Contexts of early intervention: Systems and settings* (pp. 73–92). Baltimore, MD: Brookes.

Trivette, C. M., Dunst, C. J., & Hamby, D. W. (1996). Social support and coping in families of children at risk for developmental disabilities. In M. Brambring, H. Rauh, & A. Beelmann (Eds.), *Early childhood intervention: Theory, evaluation and practice* (pp. 234–264). Berlin, Germany: de Gruyter.

Trivette, C. M., Dunst, C. J., O'Herin, C. E., & Hamby, D. W. (2008). *Meta-analysis of the influences of family strengths on parent, family and child functioning* (Winterberry Research Syntheses). Asheville, NC: Winterberry Press. (in preparation).

Zigler, E., & Berman, W. (1983). Discerning the future of early childhood intervention. *American Psychologist*, *38*, 894–906.

Zimmerman, M. A. (1990). Toward a theory of learned hopefulness: A structural model analysis of participation and empowerment. *Journal of Research in Personality*, *24*, 71–86.

Marshalling Social Support: A Care-Getting Model for Persons Living With Cancer

EVA KAHANA, BOAZ KAHANA, MAY WYKLE, and DIANA KULLE
Case Western Reserve University, Cleveland, Ohio

This article offers a stress theory–based conceptual framework for understanding proactive options for care-getting for patients living with cancer that is also relevant to patients living with other chronic or life-threatening illnesses. Barriers and facilitators to active efforts for obtaining responsive care from both informal and formal sources are discussed. This "care-getting" model explores benefits of proactive care-getting for diminishing physical discomfort and suffering, burden of illness and disability, and psychological distress. The authors highlight unique issues in care-getting that patients face at different stages of the life course. Implications of prior research related to the model for practice and intervention are discussed.

In this article, the special needs of patients as care recipients will be highlighted by focusing on challenges of patients facing serious chronic illness, as exemplified by cancer. Such illness-related challenges are not only normative for the very old but also apply to all individuals who face life-threatening illness throughout the life course. The discussion considers proactive adaptations by patients, throughout the life course, who deal with life-threatening illness such as cancer. Care-getting refers to active efforts by patients to obtain responsive care from both informal and formal

---

This research was supported by National Institutes of Health, National Cancer Institute grant RO1-CA098966.

sources. The former include family and friends, while the latter involve health care professionals. Care-getting is distinct from the commonly studied phenomenon of caregiving that describes provision of assistance, often provided by family members in the context of major illness situations. The timeliness of focusing on care-getting is underscored by the virtual absence of discourse on the challenges of care-getting among the chronically ill, despite extensive focus on issues of caregiving. Accordingly, successful care-getting may be viewed as a critical goal during a disabling illness (Wagner et al., 2001). An understanding of the maintenance of good quality of life (QOL) among chronically ill patients has been limited by the lack of systematic theoretical attention to care-getting throughout the life course. This article synthesizes orientations from the fields of sociology, social work, nursing, and psychology to expand conceptual understanding of this critical area. We build on a stress theoretical framework (Pearlin, 1989) to help appreciate the unique challenges faced by chronically ill patients. Mastery of the adaptive tasks of care-getting involves marshalling informal and formal support, which allows for obtaining the best medical care and the maintenance of comfort, psychological well-being, and a sense of being cared for (Nolan & Mock, 2004).

Even though cancer is more treatable today than in the past and the number of survivors has grown, cancer diagnosis is still one of the most feared introductions to the world of chronic and life-threatening illness (Dolbeault, Szporn, & Holland, 1999; Harpham, 1995). Patients living with cancer face uncertain futures and suffer from symptoms due to their illness as well as the treatments that they must undergo (Ng, Alt, & Gore, 2007). Indeed, treatment for cancer may involve surgery, radiation, chemotherapy, and other interventions, which carry both immediate and long-term side effects. Cancer patients may need varying levels of care during the active treatment and after-treatment phases of their illness.

Fatigue, pain, functional limitations, and emotional distress are common by-products of living with cancer (Hewitt, Greenfield, & Stovall, 2006). Given that cancer has been considered to be a highly stigmatized condition (Wolff, 2007), many cancer patients face challenges in care-getting. Many patients with cancer are reluctant to disclose the nature of their illness to friends, neighbors, and coworkers who might otherwise be natural sources of instrumental and emotional support. In terms of challenges of formal care-getting, patients must interact with a variety of specialists during their cancer experience. It is not uncommon for patients to see surgeons, medical oncologists, and radiation oncologists, in addition to follow-ups by their primary care physicians. Care-getting also poses unique challenges during the posttreatment (reentry) period, when uncertainty and ambiguity about availability of caregivers pose problems for patients (Richey & Brown, 2007).

Being diagnosed with cancer at different points during the life course presents patients with unique issues in their efforts to successfully and proactively marshal support (Kahana & Kahana, 2007a). Patients who show initiative and express assertiveness in communicating with caregivers and health care providers receive more responsive care that considers their values and preferences (Kahana & Kahana, 2007a). They may maintain control even in the face of illness, by having meaningful involvement in treatment decision making (O'Hair, Kreps, & Sparks, 2007). Our research focusing on elderly cancer patients indicated that proactivity as health care consumers is not widely practiced among the old-old (Kahana et al., in press). Nevertheless, it is noteworthy that a large proportion of elderly patients endorse proactive health care consumerism in giving advice to other cancer patients.

Features of the family structure change for individuals as they move through the life course, thereby affecting availability of caregivers (Pearlin & Zarit, 1993). The age, relationship, and resources of the most likely caregivers also shape patients' options for care-getting, as they aim to marshal informal support and responsive medical care at different stages during the life course. Focus on maintenance of the self during chronic illness underscores the abiding desire of human beings to maintain their long-established identity, retain autonomy, and garner respect from their social environment, for their values, preferences, and cultural diversity (George, 1999). Throughout much of adult life and well into healthy old age, this identity can be autonomously maintained. Being diagnosed with a serious illness such as cancer poses a challenge to this self-reliant, autonomous identity. This challenge and its successful resolution present a key adaptive task of proactive care-getting during the life course. The type of care that results in maintaining a sense of dignity while being cared for has been discussed in the work of Noddings (2003). Such care cannot be perfunctory or grudging and must reflect regard for the views and interests of the person being cared for. Autonomy and agency may be exercised by patients by taking initiatives and expressing assertiveness in order to elicit optimal care (Kahana & Kahana, 2007a).

The proactive care-getting model proposed here describes how patients can play an active role in obtaining responsive and nurturing care in dealing with life-threatening illness (Nolan & Mock, 2004). Our prior research has focused on adaptation to frailty among older adults, who are part of an ongoing longitudinal study (Kahana & Kahana, 2003a). While our discussion is informed by an in-depth understanding of care-getting in late life, we will address some of the unique issues that apply to patients at different points in the life course.

SPECIFYING THE CARE-GETTING MODEL

The proposed care-getting model for understanding the maintenance of a good QOL in the face of chronic illness is anchored in our previously articulated, proactivity-based model of successful aging (Kahana & Kahana 1996; 2003a; Figure 1). This stress theory–based model emphasizes the normative

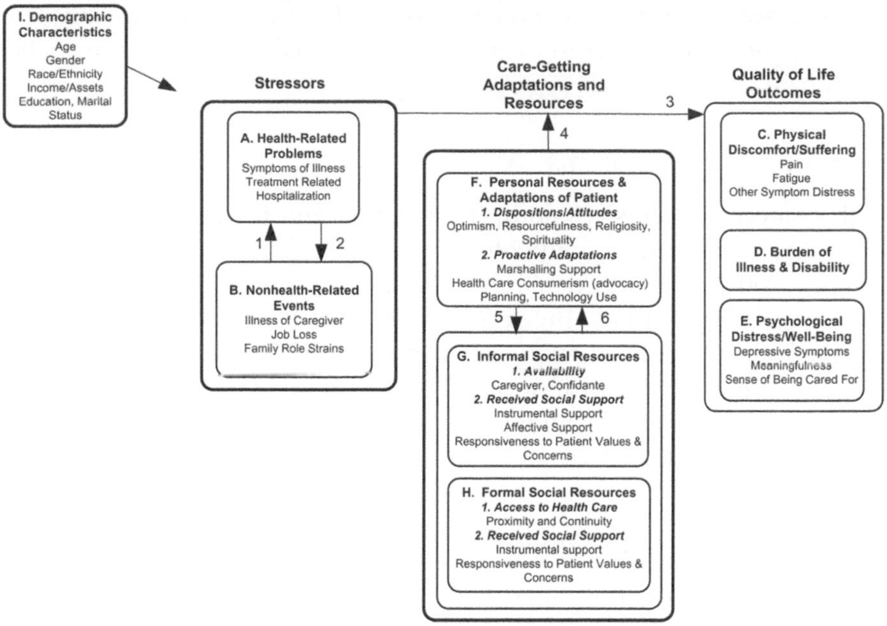

FIGURE 1 Care-Getting Model for Cancer Patients Across the Life Course.

nature of health-related stressors and social losses. It is argued that individuals must adapt proactively to ensure that they can maintain good QOL, even as they face physical impairments due to chronic illness and encounter acute health events. The care-getting model presented here emphasizes the role of proactive initiatives for using informal and formal social resources to deal with adaptive tasks of chronic illness (Moos & Schaefer, 1986). Successful care-getting helps patients secure advocates who can represent their values and wishes, even when these patients cannot do so for themselves.

The following section presents elements in the proposed model and their linkages (Figure 1). Path numbers indicate the direction of proposed causal linkages. First, antecedent stressors are described, followed by quality-of-life outcomes. We then turn to moderators, which encompass care-getting adaptations and resources and receipt of patient responsive informal and formal care. Finally, we illustrate how demographic context, representing life chances and structural constraints, may impinge on elements of the care-getting model (Giele & Elder, 1998). We also briefly describe relevant findings provided by our empirical work.

STRESSORS

Stressors are depicted as the independent variables that threaten quality-of-life outcomes (Figure 1, Components A and B). Both *health-related problems*, such as hospitalizations, and *other negative life events*, such as illness of a caregiver, are considered as they impact on the quality of the cancer patient's life (Path 3).

A. Health-related Problems

Health-related problems resulting from cancer and its treatment can disrupt functioning and result in difficult recuperation (Empana, Dargent-Molina, & Breart, 2004). Patients dealing with diverse cancers may experience a broad range of symptoms. Invasive cancer treatments ranging from surgery to chemotherapy and radiation can contribute to additional health-related problems. When hospitalization is required for symptoms or for treatment, the patient experiences additional environmental stressors that are likely to adversely impact QOL (Path 3).

B. Non-Health-Related Events

Social losses are often associated with chronic illness such as cancer, where job loss or divorce might add to the patient's sustained inability to function (Thornton & Perez, 2007). These losses can also adversely affect psychological well-being and QOL (Path 3). Patients may also face additional stressors due to illness of caregivers such as a spouse, close family members, or friends (Krause, 2006).

Health-related stressors and other critical life events may have reciprocal effects (Path 1). On the one hand, hospitalization or cancer treatments may precipitate job loss (Path 1). On the other hand, illness and unavailability of significant other caregivers could result in the need for hospitalization of the patient (Path 2).

QUALITY-OF-LIFE OUTCOMES

Three categories of quality-of-life outcomes are particularly salient in relation to chronic illness such as cancer: physical discomfort or suffering, burden of illness and disability, and psychological distress vs. well-being (Figure 1, QOL Components C, D, and E).

C. Physical Discomfort/Suffering

Physical discomfort, including pain, fatigue, and other indicators of symptom distress such as nausea, is a key component of suffering due to cancer and cancer treatments (Path 3; Cohen et al., 2005). Limiting these symptoms gains particular salience for patients with advanced disease who may be nearing the end of life (Somogyi-Zalud, Zhong, Lynn, & Hamel, 2000).

D. Burden of Illness and Disability

As seriously ill patients develop functional limitations and disability, the experience of an altered self assumes major importance (Penrod & Martin, 2003). To the extent that patients believe that they are stigmatized for their illness and feel prevented from performing important social functions, they develop negative self-evaluation and outcome expectations termed "burden of disability."

E. Psychological Distress/Well-Being

Physical symptoms and impairments reduce the psychological QOL of chronically ill patients (Path 3; Schieman & Turner, 1998). *Depressive symptoms* can result from exposure to chronic illness and critical life events (Path 3; Koenig & Blazer, 1992). A seriously ill patient who regularly experiences pain may still maintain self-esteem and escape despair by finding meaning in life (Lynn, 2000). A *sense of "being cared for"* is proposed as a unique and salient dimension of psychological well-being relevant to successful care-getting among those suffering from life-threatening illness (Watson, 2005).

CARE-GETTING ADAPTATIONS AND RESOURCES

Ameliorative resources (Figure 1, Components F, G, and H) play a moderating role in our care-getting model (Path 4). Personal resources of the patient (Component F) are reflected in psychological dispositions or attitudes and in proactive adaptations, which can help mobilize social resources (Path 5). Informal (Component G) and formal (Component H) social resources, such as access to family caregivers and to medical care, are also considered as moderators that can diminish the adverse effects of serious illness and critical life events on the individual's QOL (Antonucci, 1990). We also conceptualize social resources as potentially facilitating proactive adaptations (Path 6).

The care-getting model proposed here builds on our previously proposed proactivity model (Kahana & Kahana, 2003b) of successful aging. Proactive behaviors (e.g., helping others, planning, and marshalling support) that can position older adults for successful aging are also valuable for understanding maintenance of QOL during serious illness. It is useful to focus on adaptations that best contribute to successful care-getting from both informal and formal providers of support throughout the life course.

Personal resources reflect dispositions and attitudes that contribute to proactive behavioral adaptations. Although dispositional characteristics have been shown to be enduring (Costa & McCrae, 1990; Carver & Scheier, 1989), there is growing evidence that the environmental context may influence dispositional characteristics. The positive psychology movement has offered a new theoretical framework wherein optimism may be learned (Seligman, 1991; Peterson, 2000). Indeed, recent approaches to health promotion and coping with illness have underscored the value of cultivating positive emotions such as optimism and spirituality in order to enhance health and well-being (Fredrickson, 2000; Gillham & Reivich, 2004).

F. Personal Resources and Adaptations Promoting Care-Getting

1. Dispositions/attitudes

Optimism

Research has shown that adaptation to stressors, including those due to illness, may vary based on whether an individual has an optimistic or pessimistic life orientation (Scheier & Carver, 1985). Optimism is typically viewed as a dispositional, trait-like characteristic and has been found in prior health research to diminish distress outcomes (Facione, 2002). Optimism can thus help ameliorate adverse stress effects (Path 4). Additionally, optimistic dispositions contribute to social competence, which is needed to help marshal care and support and which can also elicit positive responses from caregivers (Path 5; Krause, 2006).

Resourcefulness

This concept has been proposed by nurse researchers as a particularly useful dispositional characteristic for coping with health-related stressors (Zausniewski, 1994). It is predicated on a belief in one's ability to cope effectively with adversity. Resourcefulness can allow for positive reframing of stressful situations, which, in turn, can result in stress inoculation during illness situations. Resourcefulness may play a useful role in care-getting and marshalling responsive care from both informal and formal providers of support (Path 5).

Religiosity

Religiosity and use of religious coping strategies are salient for coping with life-threatening illnesses (Koenig, George, & Siegler, 1988). Intrinsic religiosity may be expressed through faith, prayer, and finding meaning in religious values. Patients can draw on such religious values as they encounter illness (Moberg, 2001). Religious participation can also enhance availability of social supports based on caring interactions with church members (Krause, 2002).

Spirituality

Spirituality may be defined as having qualities of inner strength, peace, and harmony (Boswell, Kahana, & Dilworth-Anderson, 2006). Respect for patients' spiritual beliefs has been considered an important component of patient responsive care (Dane, 2004) that contributes to the maintenance of meaningfulness and personhood (Nolan & Crawford, 1997). Both religiosity and spirituality are expected to serve as buffers in the face of stressors of illness and are proposed to reduce suffering, burden of disability, and psychological distress (Path 4).

2. Proactive adaptations

Marshalling support

Marshalling support refers to actions taken by patients to mobilize available social resources (Greene, Jackson, & Neighbors, 1993). Receipt of responsive care is viewed as a function of both social resources available to patients and their propensity to disclose problems and ask for help (Charmaz, 1991). Patients generally marshal support first from informal resources, such as family and friends. The patient's life course stage is an important determinant of the types of helpers who may be available. Accordingly, children generally turn to parents, whereas adults rely on spouses or significant others, and the elderly often turn to their spouses and adult children for assistance (Pearlin, Pioli, & McLaughlin, 2001). When these efforts to marshal support from family members prove insufficient, patients may turn to health care providers and other formal sources of support (Cantor & Brennan, 2000).

Health care consumerism (advocacy)

Patients may also seek to enhance the quality of their health care through advocacy (Rodwin, 1997). Taking an active role in treatment decision making is an important aspect of maintaining control and influencing medical care when dealing with cancer and other illnesses. The growing literature on health communication emphasizes both the need for information gathering by patients and assertive health communication with formal providers to ensure responsive care (O'Hair, Kreps, & Sparks, 2007). Patients with disabilities need to be particularly assertive and creative in eliciting patient-responsive care (Path 5; Kahana & Kahana, 2001). Thus, patients in wheelchairs must show assertiveness to ensure that physicians address them rather than their caregivers. Similarly, both young and elderly patients can benefit by asking questions directly to physicians rather than accepting information relayed via a caregiver.

Planning

Planning ahead is a valuable proactive adaptation, because anticipation of future needs may reduce later problems by taking action (Soerensen & Pinquart, 2000). In taking an active role in cancer treatments, familiarity with clinical trials and making plans for alternative treatments increases patient control and options. Plans formulated prior to getting sick (including obtaining disability and long-term care insurance) can improve QOL when serious illness strikes (Wagner, Austin, & Von Korff, 1996). Patients diagnosed with cancer who may be unable to work during treatment benefit from planning for reentry into the workforce (Frank, 1995). Recently, there has also been advocacy for earlier planning for end-of-life care (Lynn, 2000). Learning about the options in one's environment can help patients familiarize themselves with available informal social resources and formal services that promote care-getting (Path 5).

Technology use

Use of technology can provide important sources of empowerment for patients as they deal with health-related challenges (Sherrod, 2006). Adolescents and young adults are increasingly adept at using the Internet for obtaining health information and socioemotional support (Zrebiec & Jacobson, 2001). Middle-aged individuals typically acquire computer skills in the workplace and can benefit from transferring these skills to coping with their illness. As new cohorts of older adults experience frailty and their mobility and life space diminish, e-mail, cell-phone use, and health-alert devices can play important roles in marshalling responsive care (Path 5; Kahana & Kahana, 2007b).

G. Informal Social Resources

1. Availability

Extensiveness of the patient's social network prior to the illness influences care-getting by creating access to informal support during illness episodes (Sarason & Sarason, 1985). Most patients prefer informal rather than formal sources of support, as they deal with illness-adaptive tasks (Moos & Schaefer, 1986). Caregivers living in the same household or nearby are more ready to provide instrumental support (e.g., help with household tasks), but even distant caregivers can help meet patients' needs (Krause, 2006). Having a confidante offers the opportunity to share concerns and solicit advice about health care issues. However, highly burdened caregivers may be less able to meet the needs of the patient (Wykle, 2005). When patients are hospitalized, having family members close by can be particularly important to enhance comfort and a sense of being cared for. Those without a social network face additional challenges in care-getting when facing a chronic illness alone (Hymovich & Hagopian, 1992).

It has long been recognized that social relationships within the informal network of the patient are affected by family dynamics. Accordingly, social interaction, particularly in the face of the crisis of illness, may become strained and characterized by conflict, particularly where a history of dysfunctional family relationships already exists (Kissane et al., 1994). In a study of women diagnosed with cancer, Bolger, Foster, Vinokur, and Ng (1996) noted that significant others who readily offered support in relation to patients' physical needs were often withholding of affective support when faced with patients' emotional distress. Thus, it is important to recognize that successful care-getting may be limited by family conflict and the ability of potential caregivers to assume supportive roles. Availability of caregiver's support refers to both physical access and emotional availability.

2. Received social support

Care-getting is fundamentally linked to *instrumental* and *affective support* from family and friends. Such support can facilitate the maintenance of good QOL, even in the face of critical events and chronic illnesses (Blanchard, Albrecht, & Ruckdeschel, 2000). When patients must deal with a new health diagnosis or treatment, the role of informal support gains importance. As hospitals increasingly discharge patients early, even when they require medical care at home, informal caregivers assume greater responsibilities. Different family members may provide alternative types of support at times of illness. For example, spouse caregivers are more likely to assist with personal tasks and report more hours of care over a longer period of time without reporting feeling burdened (Cantor & Brennan, 2000). Children and adolescents find natural caregivers in their parents. Patients who previously helped others are able to draw on willing caregivers from among friends and neighbors (Path 5; Midlarsky & Kahana, 2007). Similarly, patients who are helpful to fellow patients in hospital settings are likely to benefit from reciprocal assistance.

Responsiveness to patients' values and concerns

An important dimension of informal social resources relates to the responsiveness of family and friends to the concerns of the patient. When patients have limited control and are unable to act on their own behalf, they have a strong need to have family members heed their wishes (Otis-Green & Rutland, 2004). Seriously ill patients need family members to be their voice and work toward obtaining medical and nursing care that is consistent with their values and preferences (Cassell, 2005).

H. Formal Social Resources

1. Access to health care

Physical *proximity* to health care providers and the availability of a regular provider facilitates access to health care. As cancer patients often undergo treatment resulting in functional limitations, their access to health care may be restricted by lack of mobility and transportation. Delayed access to outpatient care results in longer hospital stays and poorer health outcomes

(Weissman, Stern, Fielding, & Epstein, 1991). During health crises, access also includes the willingness of health care providers to be contacted on short notice and respond to changing care needs of the cancer patients. Nursing professionals can play an important role in enhancing access to both care and information about self-care for cancer patients (Miaskowski et al., 2004).

2. RECEIVED SOCIAL SUPPORT

Informal and formal sources of care generally differ in the types of support provided. Formal health care providers supply mostly specialized *instrumental support*, while informal sources such as friends and family are more likely to provide emotional support. Nevertheless, during health crises, the caring and affirmation communicated by formal health care providers assumes increasing importance for the maintenance of good QOL. Informal caregivers also play a continuing instrumental role in arranging and monitoring care. Effective partnerships between informal and formal caregiving systems result in synergies that benefit both caregivers and patients (Fortinsky, 1998).

RESPONSIVENESS TO PATIENT VALUES AND CONCERNS

Patients with cancer often face treatment decisions that will have a long-term impact on their life by affecting fertility or resulting in altered body image (e.g., after mastectomy; Charmaz, 1991). Sensitivity and responsiveness of health care providers to patient preferences and concerns are beneficial in these situations. It is noteworthy that patients during different life stages and with different illness trajectories differ in preferences for information and involvement in health care decision making (Leydon et al., 2000). Health care continuity and clinician familiarity with a patient enhances responsiveness to patient preferences. Similarly, proactive articulation of values and preferences by patients also enhances responsiveness of care (Kahana & Kahana, 2001). Care in the final stages of life focuses on understanding psychological needs and providing optimal comfort to the patient.

DEMOGRAPHIC CHARACTERISTICS

Demographic characteristics of patients, such as age, gender, race or ethnicity, income, education, and marital status, impact all model elements (Figure 1). Since discussion of such influences involves a vast literature, we are limited here to providing illustrative examples. Based on the growing recognition of health disparities due to race or ethnicity and income (Geiger, 2006), we focus on illustrating racial and socioeconomic differences in illness-related stress exposure, care-getting, and QOL during illness. We expect that patients with more limited social resources will experience greater stress exposure and have more limited access to formal care. They may also be more limited in their help-seeking behaviors.

Demographic characteristics associated with more limited resources (i.e., older *age*, female *gender*, minority *race or ethnicity*, less *education*, lower *income*, and divorced or widowed *marital status*) increase the likelihood of experiencing both chronic illness and critical life events (Link & Phelan, 1995). Lack of social resources limits patients' options with regard to care-getting, particularly through reducing access to formal care. Studies have consistently found that lower socioeconomic status (SES) and minority status are related to reduced access to medical care (Kelley-Moore & Ferraro, 2004). A burgeoning literature on health care disparities reveals that members of racial minorities, including African Americans and Hispanics, are diagnosed with cancer at later stages of their illness and often lack access to state-of-the-art health care (Mor, Zinn, Angelelli, Teno, & Miller, 2004).

Availability of informal supports is influenced by demographic factors in complex ways. Members of minority groups have been shown to experience health disparities based on less access to high-quality health care but may have some advantage in obtaining informal care, as more limited social mobility of family members and stronger norms of obligation may result in family members being more available to offer care (Geiger, 2006).

Patients' attitudes toward getting medical care are also influenced by race and SES. Individuals with lower SES and limited education tend to let the doctor decide on treatment options (Scott, Shiell, & King, 1996). Furthermore, members of racial and ethnic minorities are more likely to express preferences for life-extending treatment (Leybas-Amedia, Nuno, & Garcia, 2005).

These illustrative examples provide a glimpse into the influence of sociodemographic resources on levels of stress exposure and access to care-related resources. We acknowledge the importance of both life chances and life choices (Elder & Conger, 2000) in our care-getting model. We note that equality in care-getting can be achieved only where all patients, regardless of race, class, or gender, can experience true caring in major illness situations.

CARE-GETTING THROUGH THE LIFE COURSE

The majority of research in the area of social networks and health has portrayed the relationship as static over the life course (Moren-Cross & Lin, 2006). However, the process of care-getting is dynamic, shaped by different adaptive tasks, family relationships, and illness trajectory across the life span, including childhood and adulthood (King & Elder, 1997; Moren-Cross & Lin, 2006). In the next portion of our article, we present a brief overview of issues shaping care-getting during different stages of the life course (see Table 1).

TABLE 1 Life-course Specific Care-getting Issues

Challenges to care-getting	Childhood	Adolescence	Young adulthood	Midlife	Old age
1. Personal barriers	Trust limited to parents as protectors	Embarrassed to disclose symptoms	Fearful of appearing weak and needy	Conflict between generativity needs and care-getting	Threatened by dependency when asking for help
	Unskilled in articulating needs	Negotiation skills not fully developed	Help seeking threatens independence	Illness-related loss of self-esteem limits help seeking	Unassertive in communicating needs
2. Social barriers	Wants to limit parental distress	Fears stigma from peers	Job/family responsibilities inhibit care-getting	Job/family responsibilities inhibit care-getting	Patient may also be a caregiver
3. Barriers to getting medical care	Separation from parents during treatment	Only assent required for treatment	Lack of support from partner in dealing with health care system	Lack of support from family in dealing with health care system	Comorbidities interfere with getting responsive cancer care
Facilitators of care-getting	Skillful parental advocacy and support	Strong peer support	Emotional support from partner	Emotional support from family	Advocacy by family
	Supportive school environment	e-literacy; self-advocacy	e-literacy; self-advocacy	e-literacy; self-advocacy	Patient–physician–family partnership
Issues of access/availability to formal and informal care-getting	Lack of direct communication with health care providers	Conflict with parents may inhibit medical care-getting	Availability of partner or close friends	Availability of family members friends/neighbors	Availability of spouse/adult child friends/neighbors
	Older sibling availability	Peer "shield" availability	Parent/work role strain inhibits access	Parent/work role strain inhibits access	Access to physician

Childhood

Prior literature regarding children living with cancer has focused mainly on psychological distress of family members and parents providing care to children with cancer (Svavarsdottir, 2005). It is important to understand, however, that children can play a significant role in eliciting responsive care for themselves or someone else. At this stage in life, children's ability to marshal support for themselves may be limited by absence of resources and/or constrained by parental attitudes. Given that parents are usually the primary caregivers during this life stage, marshalling support for children with cancer is shaped by responses received from their parents. In a study to evaluate the caregiving demands placed on parents of children with cancer, Svavarsdottir (2005) found that the most difficult and time-consuming activity for parents was providing emotional support.

Recognizing parents' emotional strain, children with cancer may be apprehensive to marshal additional needed support from their parents. Marshalling support from siblings can serve a useful role for children living with cancer (Kahana, Kahana, Johnson, Hammond, & Kercher, 1994). However, research has shown that the emotional toll on siblings of children with cancer is also taxing (Alderfer, Labay, & Kazak, 2003). Children with cancer must cope with isolation from normal school and social activities. Concern about physical changes distorting their body image has been found to be a prevalent issue among children with cancer (Kameny & Bearisond, 2002). Children's ability to seek and receive reassurance in these realms is an important influence on their QOL. One available option for children with cancer is the use of cancer support groups specifically geared for children. These support groups not only give needed emotional support to children suffering with cancer, but they also empower children with needed skills that can enable them to be better proactive care getters (Wright & Frey, 2007).

Parents of children with cancer must frequently allow doctors and nurses to become the caregivers (Woodgate, 1999). The child's ability to marshal support from strangers who serve as caregivers is limited, because the child may lack self-efficacy to be assertive in requesting needed care. In the case of a child with cancer, the parent–child communication dyad is typically transformed into a doctor/nurse–parent–child triad, which makes managing communication more difficult (Young, Dixon-Woods, Windridge, & Henry, 2003). Communication with children who are dealing with cancer is particularly important because it builds trust, and in turn that trust affords the child the comfort needed to be more assertive in care-getting. While adults have the ability to act as their own advocates, children in the hospital need an advocate for care-getting (Beuf, 1989). Children's age and knowledge of their illness will influence their options for self-advocacy and of marshalling support. Furthermore, children with cancer who actively seek and gather information can reduce some of their uncertainty (Husain & Moore, 2007).

Such advocacy can help decrease children's sense of isolation related to both school and family life (Wright & Frey, 2007).

Adolescence

Chronic illness, in general, and cancer, in particular, hold special challenges for adolescents. Since adolescents often have a sense of invincibility, they might deny symptoms and may be embarrassed to seek treatment early (Albritton & Bleyer, 2003). There are unique challenges to the adolescent patient who is threatened with the loss of newly won independence and who is reluctant to return to a dependent role, with parents or caregivers in charge of decision making. Part of the care-getting challenge for the adolescent diagnosed with cancer involves renegotiation of family relationships with parents and siblings.

Care-getting challenges the social development of adolescents who are eager for acceptance by their peers and threatens their ability to blend into the peer culture (Abrams, Hazen, & Penson, 2006). However, peers can become significant sources of instrumental and social support for adolescents who are able to self-disclose challenges of their illness. In terms of marshalling formal support from health care providers, adolescents are eager to be involved in decision making but often lack information about alternative options being considered (Albritton & Bleyer, 2003). Accordingly, effective proactivity as health care consumers is contingent on successful information gathering. The developmental challenges faced by adolescents to move toward greater independence from parents may serve as barriers to their ability to marshal needed instrumental, informational, and emotional support.

Adolescents also face unique challenges in care-getting from physicians, who are not required by law to obtain informed consent for treatment from patients under the age of 18. Current guidelines only require assent of adolescents in treatment (Lee, Havens, Sato, Hoffman, & Leuthner, 2006). Consequently, the ability of adolescents to obtain care that is responsive to their values and preferences may be compromised.

Studies have identified mothers as the individuals who are the major sources of social support for adolescent cancer patients. However, along with the closeness in the relationship, efforts in care-getting are often fraught with conflict, particularly in daughter–mother dyads (Marine & Miller, 1998). In addition, poor adaptation of parents and their inability to cope with the illness of their adolescent child may serve as an important barriers to successful care-getting by these young cancer patients (Frank, Blount, & Brown, 1997).

Among peers, best friends have been cited as particularly valuable in care-getting efforts of adolescent cancer patients. They can serve as "peer shields," protecting adolescents from social stigma, particularly during the reentry phase of their cancer experience, when they return to school and to their social functions (Larouche & Chin-Peuckert, 2006). With the expansion of online support groups, accessing peer-support groups can serve as a source of empowerment for young cancer patients. Alternatively, some adolescents may distance themselves from those peers with cancer.

Marshalling formal support proactively also involves taking initiative by the young patient in raising questions and concerns to a busy medical staff. Research indicates that nurses are often viewed by young patients as the most approachable health care providers (Ritchie, 2001).

Young Adulthood

Young adulthood is a period in life when important issues about personal and social identity are established within both professional and family roles. Establishment of intimate relationships with a partner represents another developmental task of young adulthood (Erikson, 1980; Levinson, 1978). Issues in marshalling support after cancer diagnosis might be particularly difficult at this stage, when the promise of a fulfilling life has just started to unfold. There has been little research dealing with young adult cancer patients in general, and specifically on care-getting, in this group. As young adults are adjusting to the transition from adolescence to adulthood and to independence, becoming a proactive care getter is particularly salient, since many of the cancers that occur during young adulthood are curable and the survival rate among this group is higher than in other age groups, including adolescence (Gatta, 2003). Nevertheless, threats to self-esteem pose challenges to care-getting, due to the "off time" nature of illness and accompanying sense of loss (Rolland, 1994).

Research on young-adult women living with breast cancer indicates that this group encounters more physical and psychosocial distress than do older women confronting this disease (Kroenke et al., 2004). These adverse effects of cancer in young adulthood have been attributed to disruption in self-image and sexuality. Disclosure of illness diagnosis necessary for marshalling informal support may also be difficult for young adults, who are likely to fear disruption of social relationships or inability to have children.

Young adults are among major users of the Internet for receiving social support online. The anonymity of online support groups allows for more comfort in discussing potentially embarrassing subjects and allows for marshalling support without revealing visible effects of treatment, such as hair loss due to chemotherapy (White & Dorman, 2001). Indeed, the term "e-patients" describes new cohorts of assertive patients who take an active role in care getting from the formal health care system (O'Hair, Kreps, & Sparks, 2007).

Midlife

Although the importance of adult life stages in the experience of cancer has been acknowledged in conceptual frameworks on cancer survivorship

(Rowland, 1989), little research has focused on unique needs and perspectives of cancer patients in midlife. Studies are largely based on age comparisons involving the young or the old, whereas middle-aged patients are often omitted from such studies (Rose et al., 2004). Being afflicted with cancer in midlife represents a major disruption in social roles related to developmental tasks of midlife, generativity (Erikson, 1993), work and family (Charmaz, 1991), and reassessment of identity (Carr, 1997).

Research focusing on age differences in coping with chronic illness in general reveals that middle-aged individuals are more likely to engage in help-seeking coping strategies than are older adults (Felton & Revenson, 1987). Interpersonal rather than self-reliant approaches may be more acceptable to younger cohorts of middle-aged patients in dealing with illness. The need for care-getting in midlife may also be viewed as being at odds with the self-image of middle-aged patients as contributing members of society. Thus, parents suffering from cancer must turn from nurturing their children to recognizing their own vulnerability and needing nurture.

Although being a recipient of care may be psychologically difficult to accept, cancer patients at midlife possess many resources that position them well for proactive care-getting. Since many adults in midlife are married, spouses represent available partners for decision making and can be readily involved in caregiving roles. Adults during midlife are at the peak of their income and careers and have the educational background to play an assertive role with health care providers. This contrasts with the greater dependency of very young and very old patients. Research on age or cohort differences among cancer patients, regarding receiving emotional support from their physicians, suggests that middle-aged patients receive more emotional support from physicians than do their elderly counterparts (Rose, 1993).

Research on midlife and chronic illness, including cancer, has often focused on the gendered nature of the illness experience. Qualitative findings have pointed to women reporting great stress, based on expectations that midlife women should fulfill work and family obligations even while undergoing debilitating treatments. When such patients feel that they do not have a voice in marshalling responsive health care, they feel overwhelmed and alienated (Kralik, 2002).

Old Age

Older adults (age 65 or over) represent a large majority of all new cases of cancer (61%), having 11 times the risk for cancer compared to younger age groups (Feuerstein, 2007). Among unique challenges faced by older adults in obtaining responsive care, barriers in communication have been noted as playing a key role. Older adults often experience sensory losses (difficulties in hearing and vision) and cognitive losses that place them at a disadvantage in expressing assertiveness and initiative in marshalling support (Sparks, 2007). Additionally, social losses (by death or relocation of family and friends) reduce access to informal sources of support in later life (Kahana & Kahana, 2003a). Based on their socialization to respect medical authority, older cancer patients have also been found to express less initiative and assertiveness in their health care encounters with physicians (Kahana et al., in press). Furthermore, based on the great value placed on self-reliance in the current generation of elders, help seeking in general may be less acceptable to this age group (Tanner, 2001). Even as we focus on disadvantages of late life in terms of access to caregivers and to the health care system, we must also note that the cancer experience appears to be less devastating to older adults than to younger patients. Older adults who are typically retired and have raised their families do not have the same degree of social role interruption, based on living with cancer, as do younger patients, who must deal with interruption of salient family and work-related roles.

With new cohorts of older adults seeking to maintain self-efficacy in late life, elders' options for playing an active role in care-getting may become more prevalent and may come to symbolize successful aging. Elderly persons of the future may develop skills in care-getting based on their midlife experiences as advocates in the course of caregiving to friends and family members (McDonald & Wykle, 2003). In this sense, caregiving and care-getting may be viewed as complementary concepts. In prior caregiving literature, the focus has often been placed on the designated caregiver, based on the diagnosed illness of a family member for whom they are responsible (Kahana & Young, 1990). Yet, in real life, both members of the elderly couple often require care, and caregiving or care-getting are a function of fluctuating health conditions of both partners. Essential elements of caring are located in the relationship between the one caring and the one being cared for (Noddings, 2003).

CONCLUSION

The proposed model of proactive care-getting represents an innovative perspective by recognizing that frailty and the need for care-getting can coexist, while still retaining agency and initiative. Individuals with chronic and life-threatening illness can still exert control over the care they get by proactively marshalling support (Kahana & Kahana, 2003b). Rather than focusing exclusively on caregiving, we believe that people can benefit from actively confronting *care-getting* issues, including advocacy, to ensure that the QOL is optimized during chronic illness experiences. Our model supports a paradigm shift toward patient empowerment, an area of sociological research that is relatively new and incomplete (Wagner et al., 2001).

The care-getting model we propose allows researchers the opportunity for empirical exploration that can help support or falsify tenets of the theory.

Patients with serious illnesses such as cancer may remain active participants in care-getting, or they may disengage and allow formal and informal social systems to define the unfolding of their journey, as they cope with their illness.

Because proactive care-getting has not been explicitly recognized to be a valued patient role, there has been little direct reference to interventions that can support or promote patients' care-getting efforts. Nevertheless, important strides have been made, particularly in the cancer care community, to offer resources that can empower and facilitate care-getting by cancer patients. The American Cancer Society offers hotlines providing access to volunteer peer counselors 24 hours a day. Accordingly, access is offered to discuss concerns and adaptive tasks faced by cancer patients. Print, audio, and online resources to support groups, focused on specific concerns and/or specific age groups, are also available through numerous patient-initiated or institutional sponsors. The "Cancer Survival Toolbox" is a particularly useful audio resource program containing 10 free CDs addressing communication skills and access to resources for survivors of different ages dealing with diverse common cancers. It is available at www.canceradvocacy.org/toolbox/. Access to relevant resources is broadly disseminated through advertising via print and broadcast media by cancer survivor organizations, including the American Cancer Society, the Lance Armstrong Foundation, the National Cancer Institute, the National Coalition for Cancer Survivorship, the Association of Oncology Social Work, and the Oncology Nursing Society. Programs to empower health care consumers to communicate more assertively and to take more initiative as patients have been limited (Epstein & Street, 2007). Nevertheless, the success of training programs for enhancing health literacy and communication competence has been reported (Cegala, Post, & McClure, 2002; Tran et al., 2004).

The proposed proactive care-getting model is aimed to generate research that is needed to support the development of future interventions. Such interventions can enhance the QOL of those dealing with the stressors associated with chronic illness. Our conceptualization holds the potential for understanding aspects of planning, health care consumerism, and marshalling social support. This will enable patients and their families to be trained to engage in and to help promote patient-responsive or patient-centered care. This can lead to interventions that empower health care consumers to take initiative and to be assertive as they manage their health care. Patient-focused interventions that foster proactive care-getting can complement educational efforts aimed at sensitizing health care providers to the special needs of patients with serious chronic illnesses such as cancer. Our focus on diverse concerns of patients with chronic illnesses, including spirituality as a resource, and meaningfulness as an outcome, can lead to culturally sensitive and humanistic interventions in the future.

REFERENCES

Abrams, A. N., Hazen, E. P., & Penson, R.T. (2006). Psychosocial issues in adolescents with cancer. *Cancer Treatment Reviews, 33*, 622–630.

Albritton, K., & Bleyer, W. A. (2003). The management of cancer in the older adolescent. *European Journal of Cancer, 39*, 2584–2599.

Alderfer, M. A., Labay, L. E., & Kazak, A. E. (2003). Brief report: Does posttraumatic stress apply to siblings of childhood cancer survivors? *Journal of Pediatric Psychology, 28*(4), 281–286.

Antonucci, T. C. (1990). Social supports and social relationships. In R. H. Binstock & L. K. George (Eds.), *Handbook of aging and the social sciences* (2nd ed., pp. 94–128). Princeton, NJ: Van Nostrand Reinhold.

Beuf, A. H. (Eds.). (1989). *Biting off the bracelet: A study of children in hospitals*; Philadelphia: University of Pennsylvania Press.

Blanchard, C. G., Albrecht, T. L., & Ruckdeschel, J. (2000). Patient-family communication with physicians. In L. Baider, C. L. Cooper, & A. K. De-Nour (Eds.), *Cancer and the family* (2nd ed., pp. 477–495). Chichester, England: John Wiley & Sons.

Bolger, N., Foster, M., Vinokur, A. D., & Ng, R. (1996). Close relationships and adjustment to a life crisis: The case of breast cancer. *Journal of Personality and Social Psychology, 70*(2), 283–294.

Boswell, G., Kahana, E., & Dilworth-Anderson, P. (2006). Spirituality and healthy lifestyle behaviors: Stress counter-balancing effects in the health maintenance of older adults. *Journal of Religion and Health.*

Cantor, M. H., & Brennan, M.. (2000). *Social care of the elderly: The effects of ethnicity, class, and culture.* New York: Springer.

Carr, D. (1997). The fulfillment of career dreams at midlife. *Journal of Health and Social Behavior, 38*, 331–344.

Carver, C. S., & Scheier, M. F. (1989). Social intelligence and personality: Some unanswered questions and unresolved issues. *Advances in Social Cognition, 2*, 93–109.

Cassell, J. (2005). *Life and death and intensive care.* Philadelphia: Temple University Press.

Cegala, D. J., Post, D. M., & McClure, L. (2002). The effects of patient communication skills training on the discourse of older patients during a primary care interview. *Journal of the American Geriatrics Society, 49*(11), 1505–1511.

Charmaz, K. (1991). *Good days, bad days: The self in chronic illness and time*; Rutgers, NJ: Rutgers University Press.

Cohen, M. Z., Musgrave, C. F., McGuire, D. B., Strumpf, N. E., Munsell, M. F., Mendoza, T. R., et al. (2005). The cancer pain experience of Israeli adults 65 years and older: The influence of pain interference, symptom severity, and knowledge and attitudes on pain and pain control. *Support Care Cancer, 13*, 708–714.

Costa, P. T., & McCrae, R. R. (1990). Personality: Another "hidden factor" is stress research. *Psychological Inquiry, 1*(1), 22–24.

Dane, B. (2004). Integrating spirituality and religion. In J. Berzoff & P. R. Silverman (Eds.), *Living with dying: A handbook for end of life health care practitioners* (pp. 424–438). New York: Columbia University Press.

Dolbeault, S., Szporn, A., & Holland, J. C. (1999) Psycho-oncology: Where have we been? Where are we going? *European Journal of Cancer, 35*(11), 1554–1558.

Elder, G. H., & Conger, R. (2000). *Children of the land: Adversity and success in rural America.* Chicago: University of Chicago Press.

Empana, J. P., Dargent-Molina, P., & Breart, G. (2004). Effect of hip fracture on mortality in elderly women: The EPIDOS prospective study. *Journal of the American Geriatrics Society, 52,* 685–690.

Epstein, R., & Street, R. (2007). *Patient-centered communication in cancer care: Promoting healing and reducing suffering* (NIH Publication No. 07–6226). Bethesda, MD: National Cancer Institute.

Erikson, E. H. (1980). *Identity and the life cycle.* New York: Norton.

Erikson, E. H. (1993). *Childhood and society.* New York: Norton.

Facione, N. C. (2002). Perceived risk of breast cancer: Influence of heuristic thinking. *Cancer Practice, 10*(5), 256–262.

Felton, B. J., & Revenson, T. (1987). Age differences in coping with chronic illness. *Psychology and Aging, 2*(2), 164–170.

Feuerstein, M. (2007). *Handbook of cancer survivorship.* New York: Springer.

Fortinsky, R. H. (1998). *Physician influence on caregivers of dementia patients.* Washington, DC: AARP.

Frank, A. (1995). *The wounded storyteller.* Chicago: University of Chicago Press.

Frank, N. C., Blount, R. L., & Brown, R. T. (1997). Attributions, coping, and adjustment in children with cancer. *Journal of Pediatric Psychology, 22*(4), 563–576.

Fredrickson, B. L. (2000). Cultivating positive emotions to optimize health and well-being. *Prevention & Treatment, 3.* Retrieved July 14, 2008 from http://journals.apa.org/prevention/volume3/toc-mar07-00.html

Gatta, G. (2003). Cancer survival in European adolescents and young adults. *European Journal of Cancer, 39*(18), 2600–2610.

Geiger, H. J. (2006). Health disparities: What do we know? What do we need to know? What should we do? In A. J. Schulz & L. Mullings (Eds.), *Gender, race, class, & health: Intersectional approaches* (pp. 261–288). San Francisco: Jossey-Bass.

George, L. K. (1999). Life-course perspectives on mental health. In C. S. Aneshensel & J. C. Phelan (Eds.), *Handbook of sociology of mental health* (pp. 565–583). Dordrecht, The Netherlands: Kluwer Academic.

Giele, J. Z., & Elder, G. H. (1998). *Methods of life course research: Qualitative and quantitative approaches.* Thousand Oaks, CA: Sage.

Gillham, J., & Reivich, K. (2004). Cultivating optimism in childhood and adolescence. *Annals of the American Academy, 591,* 146–163.

Greene, R. L., Jackson, J. S., & Neighbors, H. W. (1993). Mental health and help-seeking behavior. In J. S. Jackson, L. M. Chatters, & R. J. Taylor (Eds.), *Aging in Black America* (pp. 185–200). Newbury Park, CA: Sage.

Harpham, W. (1995). *After cancer.* New York: HarperCollins.

Hewitt, M., Greenfield, S., & Stovall, E. (2006). *From cancer patient to cancer survivor: Lost in transition*; Washington, DC: National Academies.

Husain, M., & Moore, S. (2007). Communication and childhood cancer. In D. O'Hair, G. Kreps, & L. Sparks (Eds.), *The handbook of communication and cancer care* (pp. 257–273). Cresskill, NJ: Hampton Press.

Hymovich, D. P., & Hagopian, G. A. (1992). *Chronic illness in children and adults: A psychosocial approach*. Philadelphia: Saunders.

Kahana, E., & Kahana, B. (1996). Conceptual and empirical advances in understanding aging well through proactive adaptation. In V. Bengtson (Ed.), *Adulthood and aging: Research on continuities and discontinuities* (pp. 18–41). New York: Springer.

Kahana, E., & Kahana, B. (2001). On being a proactive health care consumer: Making an "unresponsive" system work for you. *Research in Sociology of Health Care: Changing Consumers and Changing Technology in Health Care and Health Care Delivery, 19*, 21–44.

Kahana, E., & Kahana, B. (2003a). Contextualizing successful aging: New directions in age-old search. In R. Settersten, Jr. (Ed.), *Invitation to the life course: A new look at old age* (pp. 225–255). Amityville, NY: Baywood.

Kahana, E., & Kahana, B. (2003b). Patient proactivity enhancing doctor-patient-family communication in cancer prevention and care among the aged. *Patient Education and Counseling, 50*(1), 67–73.

Kahana, E., & Kahana, B. (2007a). Health care partnership model of doctor-patient communication in cancer prevention and care among the aged. In D. O'Hair, G. Kreps, & L. Sparks (Eds.), *The handbook of communication and cancer care* (pp. 37–54). Cresskill, NJ: Hampton Press.

Kahana, E., & Kahana, B. (2007b, June). *Technology use, health information, and doctor-patient communication*. Presented at the 9th World Congress of Semiotics, Helsinki/Imatra, Finland.

Kahana, E., Kahana, B., Johnson, R., Hammond, R., & Kercher (1994). Developmental challenges and family caregiving: Bridging concepts and research. In E. Kahana, D. Biegel, & M. Wykle (Eds.), *Family caregiving across the lifespan* (pp. 3–41). Thousand Oaks, CA: Sage.

Kahana, E., Kahana, B., Kelley-Moore, J., Adams, S., Hammel, R., Kulle, D., Brown, J., & King, C. (in press). Toward advocacy in cancer care among the old-old: Cautionary personal actions and bold advice to others. *Journal of American Geriatric Society*.

Kahana, E., & Young, R. (1990). Clarifying the caregiver paradigm: Challenges for the future. In D. E. Biegel & A. Blum (Eds.), *Aging and caregiving: Theory, research and practice* (pp. 76–97). Newbury Park, CA: Sage.

Kameny, R., & Bearisond, D. (2002). Cancer narratives of adolescents and young adults: A quantitative and qualitative analysis. *Children's Health Care, 31*(2), 143–173.

Kelley-Moore, J., & Ferraro, K. F. (2004). The Black/White disability gap: Persistent inequality in later life? *Journal of Gerontology: Social Sciences, 59B*, 34–43.

King, V., & Elder, G. (1997). The legacy of grandparenting: Childhood experiences with grandparents and current involvement with grandchildren. *Journal of Marriage and the Family, 59*, 848–859.

Kissane, D. W., Bloch, S., Burns, W. I., Patrick, J. D., Wallace, C. S., & McKenzie, D. P. (1994). Perceptions of family functioning and cancer. *Psycho-Oncology, 3*, 259–269.

Koenig, H. G., & Blazer, D. G. (1992). Mood disorders and suicide. In J. E. Birren, R. B. Sloane, & G. D. Cohen (Eds.), *Handbook of mental health and aging* (2nd ed., pp. 379–407). San Diego: Academic Press.

Koenig, H. G., George, L. K., & Siegler, I. C. (1988). The use of religion and other emotion-regulating coping strategies among older adults. *The Gerontologist, 28*(3), 303–310.

Kralik, D. (2002). The quest for ordinariness: Transition experience by midlife women living with chronic illness. *Journal of Advanced Nursing, 39*(2), 146–154.

Krause, N. (2002). Church-based social support and health in old age: Exploring variations by race. *The Journals of Gerontology Series B: Psychological Sciences and Social Sciences, 57*, S332–S347.

Krause, N. (2006). Social relationships in late life. In R. H. Binstock & L. K. George (Eds.), *Handbook of aging and the social sciences* (6th ed., pp. 181–200). Amsterdam, The Netherlands: Elsevier.

Kroenke, C., Rosner, B., Chen, W., Kawachi, I., Colditz, G., & Holmes, M. (2004). Functional impact of breast cancer by age. *Journal of Clinical Oncology, 22*(10), 1849–1856.

Larouche, S. S., & Chin-Peuckert, L. (2006). Changes in body image experienced by adolescents with cancer. *Journal of Pediatric Oncology Nursing, 23*(4), 200–209.

Lee, K. J., Havens, P. L., Sato, T. T., Hoffman, G. M., & Leuthner, S. R. (2006). Assent for treatment: Clinician knowledge, attitudes, and practice. *Pediatrics, 18*(2), 723–730.

Levinson, D. J. (1978). *The seasons of a man's life*. New York: Knopf.

Leybas-Amedia, V., Nuno, T., & Garcia, F. (2005). Effect of acculturation and income on Hispanic women's health. *Journal of Health Care for the Poor and Underserved, 16*, 128–141.

Leydon, G., Boulton, M., Moynihan, C., Jones, A., Mossman, J., Boudioni, M., et al. (2000). Cancer patients' information needs and information seeking behaviour: In depth interview study. *British Medical Journal, 320*, 909–913.

Link, B. G., & Phelan, J. (1995). Social conditions as fundamental causes of disease. *Journal of Health and Social Behavior, 35*, 80–94.

Lynn, J. (2000). Finding the key to reform in end of life care. *Journal of Pain and Symptom Management, 19*(3), 165–167.

Marine, S., & Miller, D. (1998). Social support, social conflict, and adjustment among adolescents with cancer. *Journal of Pediatric Psychology, 23*(2), 121–130.

McDonald, P. E., & Wykle, M. L. (2003). Predictors of health-promoting behavior of African-American and White caregivers of impaired elders. *Journal of National Black Nurses Association, 14*(1), 1–12.

Miaskowski, C., Dodd, M., West, C., Schumacher, K., Paul, S. M., Tripathy, D., et al. (2004). Randomized clinical trial of the effectiveness of self-care intervention to improve cancer pain management. *Journal of Clinical Oncology, 22*, 1713–1720.

Midlarsky, L., & Kahana, E. (2007). Life course perspectives on altruistic health and mental health. In S. Post (Ed.), *Altruism and health: Perspectives from empirical research* (pp. 81–103). New York: Oxford University Press.

Moberg, D. O. (2001). The reality and centrality of spirituality. In D. O. Moberg (Ed.), *Aging and spirituality* (pp. 3–20). New York: Haworth Pastoral Press.

Moos, R., & Schaefer, J. (1986). Life transitions and crises: A conceptual overview. In R. H. Moos (Ed.), *Coping with life crisis: An integrated approach* (pp. 3–28). New York: Plenum Press.

Mor, V., Zinn, J., Angelelli, J., Teno, J., & Miller, S. (2004). Driven to tiers: Socio-economic and racial disparities in the quality of nursing home care. *The Milbank Quarterly, 82*, 227–256.

Moren-Cross, J., & Lin, N.. 2006. Social networks and health. In R. H. Binstock & L. K. George (Eds.), *Handbook of aging and the social sciences* (6th ed., pp. 111–126). San Diego: Elsevier.

Ng, A. V., Alt, C. A., & Gore, E. M. (2007). Fatigue. In M. Feuerstein (Ed.), *Handbook of cancer survivorship* (pp. 133–150). New York: Springer.

Noddings, N. (2003). *Caring: A feminine approach to ethics and moral education* (2nd ed.). Berkeley: University of California Press.

Nolan, P., & Crawford, P. (1997). Towards a rhetoric of spirituality in mental health care. *Journal of Advanced Nursing, 26*, 289–294.

Nolan, M. T., & Mock, V. (2004). A conceptual framework for end of life care: A reconsideration of factors influencing the integrity of the human person. *Journal of Professional Nursing: Official Journal of the American Association of Colleges of Nursing, 20*(6), S351–S360.

O'Hair, D., Kreps, G., & Sparks, L. (2007). Conceptualizing cancer care and communication. In D. O'Hair, G. Kreps, & L. Sparks (Eds.), *The handbook of communication and cancer care* (pp. 1–12). Cresskill, NJ: Hampton Press.

Otis-Green, S., & Rutland, C. B. (2004). Marginalization at the end of life. In J. Berzoff & P. R. Silverman (Eds.), *Living with dying: A handbook for end of life health care practitioners* (pp. 462–481). New York: Columbia University Press.

Pearlin, L. (1989). The sociological study of stress. *Journal of Health and Social Behavior, 30*, 241–257.

Pearlin, L., Pioli, M., & McLaughlin, A. (2001). Caregiving by adult children: Involvement, role disruption, and health. In R. H. Binstock & L. K. George (Eds.), *Handbook of aging and the social sciences* (5th ed., pp. 238–253). San Diego: Academic Press.

Pearlin, L., & Zarit, S. (1993). Research into informal caregiving: Current perspectives and future directions. In S. H. Zarit, L. I. Pearlin, & K. W. Schaie (Eds.), *Caregiving systems: Informal and formal helpers* (pp. 155–167). Hillsdale, NJ: Lawrence Earlbaum.

Penrod, J., & Martin, P. (2003). Health expectancy, risk factors, and physical functioning. In L. W. Poon, S. H. Gueldner, & B. M. Sprouse (Eds.), *Successful aging and adaptation with chronic diseases* (pp. 104–115). New York: Springer.

Peterson, C. (2000). The future of optimism. *American Psychologist, 55*(1), 44–55.

Richey, J., & Brown, J. (2007). Cancer, communication, and the social construction of self: Modeling the construction of self in survivorship. In D. O'Hair, G. Kreps, & L. Sparks (Eds.), *The handbook of communication and cancer care* (pp. 145–164). Cresskill, NJ: Hampton Press.

Ritchie, M. A. (2001). Sources of emotional support for adolescents with cancer. *Association of Pediatric Hematology/Oncology Nurses, 18*(3), 105–110.

Rodwin, M. A. (1997). The neglected remedy: Strengthening consumer voice in managed care. *The American Prospect, 34*(9–/10), 45–50.

Rolland, J. S. (1994). *Families, illness, and disability: An integrative treatment model*; New York: Basic Books.

Rose, J. (1993). Interactions between patients and providers: An exploratory study of age differences in emotional support. *Journal of Psychosocial Oncology, 11*(2), 43–67.

Rose, J. H., O'Toole, E. E., Dawson, N. V., Lawrence, R., Gurley, D., Thomas, C., et al. (2004). Perspectives, preferences, care practices, and outcomes among older and middle-aged patients with late-stage cancer. *Journal of Clinical Oncology, 22*(24), 4907–4917.

Rowland, J. H. (1989). Developmental stage and adaptation: Adult model. In J. C. Holland & J. H. Rowland (Eds.), *Handbook of psycho-oncology* (pp. 25–43). Oxford, UK: Oxford University Press.

Sarason, I. G., & Sarason, B. R. (1985). *Social support: Theory, research, and applications.* Boston: Martinus Nijhoff.

Scheier, M., & Carver, C. (1985). Optimism, coping, and health: Assessment and implications of generalized outcome expectancies. *Health Psychology, 4*, 219–247.

Schieman, S., & Turner, H. A. (1998). Age, disability, and the sense of mastery. *Journal of Health and Social Behavior, 39*(3), 169–186.

Scott, A., Schiell, A., & King, M. (1996). Is general practitioner decision making associated with patient socio-economic status? *Social Science & Medicine, 42*(1), 35–46.

Seligman, M. E .P. (1991). *Learned optimism*. New York: Knopf.

Sherrod, R. A. (2006). Nursing research: Improving interest and understanding for the Net Generation. *Nurse Educator, 31*(2), 49–52.

Soerensen, S., & Pinquart, M. (2000). Vulnerability and access to resources as predictors of preparation for future care needs in the elderly. *Journal of Aging and Health, 12*(3), 275–300.

Somogyi-Zalud, E., Zhong, Z., Lynn, J., & Hamel, M. B. (2000). Elderly persons' last six months of life: Findings from the hospitalized elderly longitudinal project. *Journal of the American Geriatrics Society, 48*(5), 131–139.

Sparks, L. (2007). Cancer care and the aging patient: Complexities of age-related communication barriers. In D. O'Hair, G. L. Kreps, & L. Sparks (Eds.), *The handbook of communication and cancer care* (pp. 227–244). Cresskill, NJ: Hampton Press.

Svavarsdottir, E. K. (2005). Caring for a child with cancer: A longitudinal perspective. *Journal of Advanced Nursing, 50*(2), 153–161.

Tanner, D. (2001). Sustaining the self in later life: Implications for community-based services. *Ageing and Society, 21*(3), 255–278.

Thornton, A. A., & Perez, M. A. (2007). Interpersonal relationships. In M. Feuerstein (Ed.), *Handbook of cancer survivorship* (pp. 191–210). New York: Springer.

Tran, A., Haidet, P., Street, R., O'Malley, K., Martin, F., & Ashton, C. (2004). Empowering communication: A community-based intervention for patients. *Patient Education & Counseling, 52*, 113–121.

Wagner, E. H., Austin, B. T., Davis, C., Hindmarsh, M., Schaefer, J., & Bonomi, A. (2001). Improving chronic illness care: Translating evidence into action. *Health Affairs, 20*(6), 64–78.

Wagner, E. H., Austin, B. T., & Von Korff, M. (1996). Organizing care for patients with chronic illness. *The Milbank Quarterly, 74*(4), 511–544.

Watson, J. (2005). *Caring science as sacred science*; Philadelphia: F. A. Davis.

Weissman, J. S., Stern, R., Fielding, S. L., & Epstein, A. M. (1991). Delayed access to health care: Risk factors, reasons, and consequences. *Annals of Internal Medicine, 114*(4), 325–331.

White, M., & Dorman, S. (2001). Receiving social support online: Implications for health education. *Health Education Research, 16*(6), 693–707.

Wolff, S. (2007). The burden of cancer survivorship: A pandemic of treatment success. In M. Feuerstein (Ed.), *Handbook of cancer survivorship* (pp. 7–18). New York: Springer.

Woodgate, R. (1999). Social support in children with cancer: A review of the literature. *Journal of Pediatric Oncology Nursing, 16*(4), 201–213.

Wright, K., & Frey, L. (2007). Communication and support groups for people living with cancer. In D. O'Hair, G. Kreps, & L. Sparks (Eds.), *The handbook of communication and cancer care* (pp. 37–54). Cresskill, NJ: Hampton Press.

Wykle, M. L. (2005). Health and productivity—challenging the mystique of longevity. In M. L. Wykle, D. L. Morris, & P. J. Whitehouse (Eds.), *Successful aging through the lifespan: Intergenerational issues in health*. New York: Springer.

Young, B., Dixon-Woods, M., Windridge, K., & Henry, D. (2003). Managing communication with young people who have a potentially life threatening chronic illness: Qualitative study of patients and parents. *British Medical Journal, 326*(8), 326–305.

Zausniewski, J. A. (1994). Health-seeking resources and adaptive functioning in depressed and nondepressed adults. *Archives of Psychiatric Nursing, 8*, 159–168.

Zrebiec, J. F., & Jacobson, A. M. (2001). What attracts patients with diabetes to an Internet support group? A 21–month longitudinal website study. *Diabetic Medicine, 18*(2), 154–158.

Characteristics and Trends in Family-Centered Conceptualizations

PAMELA EPLEY
Erikson Institute, Chicago, Illinois

JEAN ANN SUMMERS and ANN TURNBULL
University of Kansas, Lawrence, Kansas

Early-intervention and early childhood professionals have long considered family-centered service delivery best practice. Exactly what family-centered practice means, however, remains unclear. The lack of consensus in defining family centeredness results in incongruence in the manner and degree to which professionals implement family centeredness. This review of the literature examines current conceptualizations of family-centered practice in an effort to determine whether there is a common definition; and, if so, how that definition has changed over the past decade. The authors found that, though the key elements of family centeredness (i.e., family as the unit of attention, family choice, family strengths, family–professional relationship, and individualized family services) have remained consistent, the emphasis has shifted from the family as the unit of attention to family–professional relationship and family choice. Implications for early intervention practice and research are discussed.

The concept of family-centered practice made an appearance in discussions about early intervention (EI) and early childhood special education (ECSE) in the early 1980s (Dunst, Trivette, & Deal, 1988; Shelton, Jeppson, & Johnson, 1989; Turnbull, Summers, & Brotherson, 1984). Since then, it has become an integral principle guiding the design and delivery of service models (Bailey,

2001; Blue-Banning, Summers, Frankland, Nelson, & Beegle, 2004; Bruder, 2000; Hebbeler et al., 2007; McWilliam, Snyder, Harbin, Porter & Munn, 2000; Turnbull, Summers, Lee, & Kyzar, 2007) and personnel development (Granlund & Bjorck-Akesson, 2000; McWilliam, Tocci, & Harbin, 1998; Nelson, Summers & Turnbull, 2004). Since 1993, the Division of Early Childhood (DEC) has recognized family-centered practice as the recommended model of service delivery for EI (McWilliam & Strain, 1993; Odom & McLean, 1993; Vincent & Beckett, 1993). DEC currently characterizes family centeredness as a philosophy and practice that recognizes the centrality and enhances the strengths and capabilities of families who have children with disabilities (Trivette & Dunst, 2005).

The 1986 reauthorization of the Individuals with Disabilities Education Act (IDEA) embodied principles of family-centered practice in many ways. Congress established the Program for Infants and Toddlers with Disabilities (Part C of IDEA) in recognition of, among other things, "an urgent and substantial need . . . to enhance the capacity of families to meet the special needs of their infants and toddlers with disabilities" (Education of All Handicapped Children Act, 1986, 1431(a)(4)). With the addition of Part C, IDEA authorized services to infants and toddlers with disabilities and their families for the first time. Moreover, by creating and requiring individualized family service plans (as opposed to Individualized Education Plans), Congress made explicit the expectation that EI provide supports and services to families of young children with disabilities. Advocates for families at the time hailed this policy as an important step forward for serving families and young children (Shelton et al., 1989).

A decade later, Allen and Petr (1996) maintained that "despite its broad use, the term *family-centered* still causes confusion because it is used by authors in different ways" (p. 58). In an effort to clarify the definition, Allen and Petr reviewed definitions of *family centered* across the disciplines of social work, health, and education. Based on a content analysis of 28 definitions in more than 120 peer-reviewed articles, Allen and Petr derived the following definition to reflect thinking of family centered across disciplines: "*Family-centered service delivery*, across disciplines and settings, views the family as the unit of attention. This model organizes assistance in a collaborative fashion and in accordance with each individual family's wishes, strengths, and needs" (p. 64). The list that follows identifies the six key elements of family centeredness and the percentage of articles they reviewed that included each of the elements: family as the unit of attention (100%), family choice (29%), family strengths (25%), family–professional relationship (36%), family needs (32%), and individualized services (32%). Family as the unit of attention is described as focus on the family with the recognition that children cannot be adequately served without considering the needs of their families. The entire family, therefore, "becomes a focus of assessment, planning, and intervention, even though the presenting concern may relate to only a part of the family" (p. 64). *Family choice* referred to the organization and provision of services in accordance to families' wishes and choices. In family-centered service delivery, families are, whenever possible, "the primary and ultimate directors of and decision makers in the caregiving process" (p. 65). *Family strengths* were defined as acknowledging, incorporating, and building upon the family strengths. Empowerment of families was also associated with the element of family strengths. *Family–professional relationship* was described as family members and professionals in equal partnership and included such concepts as equality, mutuality, and teamwork. The element of family needs entailed services offered and available to all family members with a holistic view of families' "circumstances, concerns, and resources" (p. 65). Last, *individualized services* referred to assessment, goal setting, and interventions matched to the needs of each family.

Now, more than 20 years after the establishment of Part C services for infants and toddlers with disabilities and their families, the literature continues to include concerns about shortfalls in the full implementation of family-centered practice (Bruder, 2000; Campbell & Halbert, 2002; Murray & Mandell, 2004, 2006; Parette & Brotherson, 2004; Turnbull, Summers, Turnbull et al., 2007). Although policy and professional guidelines endorse family centeredness, researchers (Soodak & Erwin, 2000) and anecdotal accounts (Bruder, 2000; Lea, 2006; Rao, 2000) describe recent examples of parents' difficulties in forming partnerships with EI and early childhood professionals. Based on an analysis of Part C state-reported data, Turnbull, Summers, Turnbull et al. (2007) found that, though the percentage of families receiving family-focused services declined from 1994 to 2001, the percentage of families receiving child-focused services increased. Furthermore, research on parents' perceptions of EI services also indicates a greater satisfaction with child- than family-focused services (Bailey, Scarborough, Hebbeler, Spiker, & Mallik, 2004; Hebbeler et al., 2007) and a gap between the services and supports families receive and what they believe they need (Summers et al., 2007; Turnbull, Summers, Turnbull et al., 2007). These data raise questions about the provision of family-centered practice in EI.

The purpose of this review was to examine (1) whether conceptualizations of family-centered practice have changed over the last decade and (2) whether there is currently a commonly understood definition. A clear understanding of how *family-centered practice* is defined in the literature is important for several reasons. First, it provides a starting point for reaching consensus among researchers, professionals, policy makers, and families about the meaning of family centeredness. Second, a clear understanding of family-centered practice provides guidance for a common set of competencies for professionals, curricula for professional development, and standards for programs related to serving and supporting families. Finally, it provides a basis for evaluating the implementation and outcomes of family-centered practice. In this article, we (1) describe our method and framework for analysis, (2) present findings regarding the key elements currently included in definitions of *family-centered practice*, and (3) discuss implications for EI research.

METHOD

Search Process

To perform a comprehensive review of the literature on family-centered practice across the disciplines of education, social work, and health, we conducted computer searches of ERIC, psychINFO, Wilson Web, and Educator's Reference Complete Database for articles published between 1996 and 2007. Keywords for the natural language search included *famil** and *cent** (truncated to include all forms of the terms). Controlled language search terms included *families, disabilities, early intervention, parent-teacher relationships*, and *young children*. We then reviewed abstracts of articles matching the search terms and eliminated articles unrelated to early intervention, early childhood education, or the provision of services to children with disabilities or their families. Our initial search yielded a total of 177 articles. We evaluated articles for inclusion in this review using three preliminary criteria: the article was published in a peer-reviewed journal between 1996 and 2007, reported original research or perspective, and included a constitutive or operational definition of *family centered*. We excluded unpublished articles, doctoral dissertations, and presentations. Seventy-seven articles met these criteria. We then excluded seven response articles to Mahoney et al. (1999) and two responses to Bailey (2001) that responded to but did not necessarily present an original perspective. Of the remaining 68 articles, we excluded five that did not explicitly define *family-centered practice*. Although these five articles contained references to and descriptions of family-centered practice, we were unable to identify a specific definition that did not include our own interpretation and potential bias.

Coding

Examining the six elements of family-centered practice identified by Allen and Petr (1996), we found considerable overlap in the definitions and descriptions of family needs and individualized services. The component of family needs, for example, is described as family-centered services that take into account the "family's circumstances, concerns, and resources" (p. 65) and allows for changes in family's needs. Individualized services, on the other hand, are referred to as services matched to meet the needs and resources of each family. Due to the similarities inherent in these two elements, we combined family needs and individualized services. We then used the following five key elements as a framework for analyzing current definitions of family centeredness: (1) family as the unit of attention, (2) family choice, (3) family strengths, (4) family–professional relationship, and (5) individualized family services.

For purposes of accuracy and reliability, the senior author coded each article on two separate occasions within a time span of 2 weeks. Examples of items coded as family as the unit of attention include "family orientation" and "meet the needs of the entire family." Definitions of *family-centered practice* that included "family control" and "parental decision making" were coded as family choice. We coded phrases such as "strengths-based perspective," "empowered and enabled" families, "promoting family capabilities and capacities," and "strengthening family function" as family strengths. References to trust, respect for cultural diversity, and collaborative relationships were coded as family–professional relationship. Finally, examples of individualized family services include parent training, service coordination, support groups, and respite care. To assess reliability of coding, the second author randomly selected, read, and coded 25% of the articles using the same coding system as the primary investigator. Coding was consistent across coders at 95% with differences not being of a substantive nature.

FINDINGS

In reviewing the literature on family-centered practice, our intention was to examine current conceptualizations of family-centered practice and determine how conceptualizations may have changed over the past decade. Consequently, we evaluated current definitions for the presence of the five key elements of family centeredness: family as the unit of attention, family choice, family strengths, family–professional relationship, and individualized family services. Comparing the presence of these elements in the education, social work, and heath literature, we found no substantial differences. Therefore, this section presents current conceptualizations of family-centered practice across all three fields.

Family as the Unit of Attention

In analyzing current conceptualizations of family-centered practice, we first examined the element family as the unit of attention. In addressing the family as a whole, family-centered service delivery recognizes that "children cannot be served appropriately without consideration of the family or families with whom they [live]" (Allen & Petr, 1996, p. 64). Therefore, to the extent necessary, assessments, Individualized Family Service Plan (IFSP) development, and interventions must focus on the concerns and needs of the entire family (Allen & Petr). Of the 63 articles reviewed, nearly two thirds specifically defined *family centeredness* as treating the family as the unit of attention. Although wording varied somewhat within articles, we considered a focus on families' needs, improving family quality of life and well-being, and individualized family support and outcomes consistent with the concept of family as the unit of attention.

Other characterizations of families as the unit of attention included viewing the family holistically (Erickson, Hatton, Roy, Fox, & Renne, 2007; Farmer, Clark, & Marien, 2003) and recognizing the family as the client (Guillett, 2002; Hamilton, Roach, & Riley, 2003; King, Rosenbaum, & King, 1997). Several definitions of *family centeredness* referred explicitly to meeting the needs of families unrelated to their child with a disability (Crais, Roy, & Free, 2006; Cress, 2004; McWilliam et al., 2000). McWilliam, Snyder, Harbin, Porter, and Munn (2000), for example, described *family centeredness* as, in part, attending to family concerns "whether or not related to the child" (p. 520). Moreover, Herman (2007), Larsson (1999), and Parette and Brotherson (2004) made specific reference to parent and family outcomes in addition to child outcomes.

Family Choice

The second element of family-centered practice is family choice. Allen and Petr (1996) argued that family centeredness maximizes family choice in defining one's family, making decisions regarding service delivery, determining the nature of family–professional relationships, controlling confidentiality and sharing of information, and identifying primary concerns and goals. Of the articles reviewed, approximately three-fourths identified family choice as an element of family centeredness, often identified verbatim. Other frequent descriptions of family choice included family decision making and collaboration in identifying goals, practices, and interventions. Operational definitions included family control over services/resources and families taking control over their lives.

Although we identified family choice in a large majority of articles, we also noted marked differences in the degree or extent of choice. Family choice ranged from parents as ultimate decision makers to collaborators in goal setting. Of the 63 articles reviewed, 10 identified families as the ultimate or key decision makers in a family-centered service delivery model. King et al. (1997), for example, asserted that parents have "ultimate control over decision making" (p. 41). Similarly, Fox, Dunlap, and Cushing (2002) described parental "control over where, when, and how the services will be provided and implemented" (p. 150). Although Herman (2007) did not explicitly convey ultimate parental control, he similarly described parental decision-making powers regarding all child services and interventions.

More commonly, conceptualizations of family choice emphasized parental involvement rather than ultimate choice in decision making. Nearly one third of articles identifying family choice as an element of family centeredness described parents as partners in decisions regarding EI. We found frequent references to parents' shared responsibility in making decisions regarding EI practices, goals, services, and interventions. Examples of shared decision making include parents as partners in making decisions (Farmer et al., 2003; Gallagher, Rhodes, & Darling, 2004; Koller, Nicholas, Goldie, Gearing, & Selkirk, 2006) and "family-driven decision-making" (Starble, Hutchins, Favro, Prelock, & Bitner, 2005, p. 48).

Although Allen and Petr (1996) conceptualized family choice across multiple dimensions, we found choice predominantly associated with decisions regarding identification of needs and concerns, appropriate interventions, and service delivery. Family choice was less frequently associated with the nature and extent of the family–professional partnership, families' level of participation and decision making, defining one's family, and information sharing. Of the articles identifying family choice as a key element of family-centered practice, we found mention of choice concerning the family–professional partnerships and level of parental participation only twice. What is more, we failed to find reference of family choice concerning defining one's family or how and with whom information is shared.

Family Strengths

Family strengths, the third key element in the analysis of family centeredness, entail a commitment to and respect for the strengths and capabilities of each family member (Allen & Petr, 1996). This means not only considering family strengths, but also "incorporating them into intervention plans, and building upon them" (p. 65). This requires a change in how family members are perceived—from causes of problems and barriers to collaborative partners with positive attributes, abilities, and resources (Allen & Petr, 1996).

We identified family strengths as a component of family-centered practice in approximately one half the articles. References included a strengths-based perspective and acknowledging, promoting, or focusing on child and family strengths. Descriptions such as empowering and enabling families, enhancing families' capabilities and competencies, strengthening family functioning, and recognizing the unique qualities in each family were also consistent with the element of family strengths. In addition to recognizing and building upon family strengths, McWilliam and colleagues (McWilliam et al., 1998; McWilliam et al., 2000) called attention to another aspect of strengths-based perspective: enhancing families' confidence and belief in their own abilities. This reflected Allen and Petr's (1996) assertion that identification of strengths and opportunities for choice are intertwined. A belief in families' strengths and decision-making capabilities by families and providers maximizes family choice and their sense of competency. Although slightly more than one half the articles recognized family strengths as a component of family-centered practice, only McWilliam and colleagues (McWilliam et al., 1998; McWilliam et al., 2000) included building families' awareness and confidence in their strengths into a strengths-based perspective. While Koller et al. (2006) and Trivette and Dunst (2004) proposed family centeredness as a means of enhancing families' feelings of competency and confidence, they do so within the context of effective family–professional relationships rather than as a component of a strengths-based perspective.

Family–Professional Relationship

Family–professional relationship generally refers to the partnership between families and professionals. We found family–professional relationship in 90% of the definitions of *family-centered practice*. Collaborative partnerships, cultural responsiveness, information sharing, and "help-giving" practices were commonly cited examples of successful family–professional relationships. Respectfulness and sensitivity to families' needs, honesty, developing mutual trust, listening, and understanding families' perspectives were also noted. Other noteworthy examples of positive family–professional relationship included giving parents an optimistic view of the future (Bailey et al., 1998), offering families a sense of hopefulness by emphasizing strengths and progress (Cress, 2004; Winton & Bailey, 1997), and professional flexibility (Dunst & Bruder, 2002; Herman, 2007; Nelson et al., 2004; Starble et al., 2005). Collectively, these conceptualizations illustrate how EI providers develop relationships with and respond to many families' concerns and needs through successful family–professional relationships.

Individualized Family Services

The final element we examined in definitions of *family-centered practice* was individualized family services. Family services that are individualized match the needs and resources of each individual family (Allen & Petr, 1996). Of the articles reviewed, almost one half mentioned family-focused services to meet specific family needs. These encompassed services led by families and those led by professionals. Cited most frequently were services led by families such as Parent to Parent support. The most commonly noted professionally-led services included service coordination, parent training, information, and education. Less frequently noted family services provided by professionals were respite care, family counseling, and professionals accompanying families to meetings and appointments.

References to other family services were limited or isolated. Bodner-Johnson (2001) and Hamilton et al. (2003), for example, discussed social and recreational activities for families. Additionally, Fox et al. (2002) and Truesday-Kennedy, McConkey, Ferguson, and Roberts (2006) referred to person-centered planning for families. Only two articles, Mahoney and

Bella (1998) and Ridgley and Hallam (2006), referred to financial assistance. Last, Nelson et al. (2004) alone noted transportation as a family service.

DISCUSSION

The purpose of this review was to examine current family-centered conceptualizations to determine whether there has been a change in recent years and if there is a commonly understood current definition. We draw themes from the data to address these two purposes, identify implications for EI research, and highlight limitations of this review.

Past and Current Conceptualizations of Family-Centered Practice

The key elements of family-centered practice identified a decade ago remain fundamental to current conceptualizations. The emphases, however, appears to have changed. The element of the family as the unit of attention has decreased; family choice, family strengths, and family relationships have increased, and family services has stayed about the same. Allen and Petr (1996) identified the family as the unit of attention as the most frequently emphasized element; whereas the current element most frequently emphasized is family–professional relationship. Although we have no data that directly addresses the reason for the decreased emphasis on the family as the unit of attention, we conjecture that this decrease is consistent with an overall downward trend from 1994 to 2001 in the percentage of families who receive family-related supports and services in EI programs. Overall data on child and family services have indicated a downward trend for family services and an upward trend for child services (Danaher & Armijo, 2005). These findings and other related data on trends in providing services and supports to families of children during the early childhood years indicate that the major emphasis over the last decade has been on how families are treated (family choice, family relationship) as contrasted to what services are offered (Turnbull, Summers, Turnbull, et al., 2007). The trends reported in this article in terms of the decrease in family as the unit of attention also suggest a decrease in who in the family receives services. Clearly family support programs delivered through early childhood programs are heavily focused on mothers as the sole family member of family intervention (Friend, Summers, & Turnbull, 2009).

Extent of a Commonly Understood Definition of *Family-Centered Practice*

Based on our data, given that 90% of the articles address family–professional relationship, we can confirm that this element is commonly accepted. Three other elements have a midrange extent of acceptance: family choice, family as the unit of attention, and family strengths. Given that only one third of the articles address individualized family services as an aspect of family-centered service, we conclude that this element is not commonly accepted.

We find the lack of inclusion of individualized family services as part of the definition of *family-centered practice* especially problematic. Federal data based on EI services identified on IFSPs indicates increased child services and decreased family services over the past decade (National Early Childhood Technical Assistance Center, 2004). Moreover, research shows greater parental satisfaction with child- versus family-related services (Bailey et al., 2004; Summers et al., 2007). Collectively, the low emphasis on individualized family services in this review and these findings on decreased family services and lower parental satisfaction with family-related services support the recent view that EI has focused primarily on how professionals support families (through collaborative relationships) but has not sufficiently addressed what supports and services should be available (Turnbull, Summers, Turnbull et al., 2007). Turnbull, Summers, Turnbull et al. (2007) suggested that one reason the field of early childhood has failed to develop a conceptual framework for what resources families should receive goes back to the emphasis on family choice and reluctance to prescribe a "menu" of supports and services. They argued, however, that families and providers often lack information on appropriate or available supports and services and maintain "people cannot exercise choice if they do not know what their choices are" (p. 188).

The lower emphasis on family services is also consistent with the Office of Special Education Programs' (OSEP) recently adopted family outcomes for Part C. Despite recommendations by the Early Childhood Outcomes Center (ECO) that family outcomes include having support systems and being able to access community services, EI programs are only responsible for parents (1) knowing their rights, (2) being able to effectively communicate their child's needs, and (3) being able to help their child develop and learn (Bailey et al., 2006). OSEP declined to adopt outcomes more directly related to family services. If EI and early childhood programs are to effectively meet the needs of children with disabilities and families, family-centered practice must address services for children and families that enhance child and family outcomes. It is essential to have positive family–professional relationships, family as the unit of attention, family choice, and family strengths; however, the provision of specific family-focused services is necessary and appropriate.

Implications for EI Practice and Research

We suggest three implications from this review of family-centeredness conceptualizations for future research. First, we suggest that it would be efficacious if national family organizations and professional organizations across disciplines involved in the delivery of EI/early childhood services would partner in explicating key essential elements of family centeredness (Turnbull, Summers, Lee, et al., 2007). Our analysis of explicating definitions from published literature inherently depends primarily on professional perspectives concerning key components. Thus, our recommendation of family organizations and professional leaders partnering is to ensure a strong family voice in delineating key components and to establish consensus across disciplines. We think it is especially important, in light of societal economic circumstances with the corresponding cutbacks of programs that are occurring, to reach strong consensus on the key elements of family centeredness and then to advocate strongly for the full implementation of the agreed-upon elements. Once consensus is reached on elements, we also suggest that family and professional organizations work together to establish key indicators of each element and rubrics that professionals and families can use to document the extent to which all elements are incorporated in professional development and service delivery.

Second, once there is strong consensus on the key elements of family centeredness across family and professional communities, there is a critical need for research to investigate means of effectively preparing early childhood professionals' implementation of family-centered practice. Such research has implications for professional development, continuing education, administrative structures of early childhood programs, and program assessment. McCormick, Vail, and Gallagher (2002) stated that the "behaviors, competencies, and skills required in the provision of services to infants and toddlers and their families are qualitatively different from those typically included in programs preparing personnel to work with preschool or school-aged children" (p. 299). One particular difference is the need for interdisciplinary efforts and partnerships. Fortunately, programs specifically designed to prepare students for family-centered practice have been found to be effective and result in graduates using more family-centered practices (Pretti-Frontczak, Giallourakis, Janas, & Hayes, 2002). Research suggests that increased quantity and variety of interactions with families during in-service training improves graduates' understanding and implementation of family-centered practices (Mandell & Murray, 2005). We especially endorse the approach to research carried out by Murray and Curran (2008) in which they use mixed methods to compare nontraditional and traditional approaches to teaching family-centered values and practices to undergraduate students. The superiority of their nontraditional approach to having family members team teach with university faculty and having parents of children with disabilities participating in the course with undergraduate students provides innovative approach to building competencies. We recommend replication of the research that has been conducted documenting the positive outcomes of using a family-centered approach to teach family centeredness.

Third, a significant need for future research is focusing on the outcomes of family-centered processes. Allen and Petr (1996) noted the interest by families, policy makers, and program funders in the correlation between family-centered practice and outcomes of services over a decade ago. Interest in the relationship between services and outcomes remains paramount. Although not specifically focused on outcomes of family-centered practice, the National Early Intervention Longitudinal (NEILS) Study (Bailey et al., 2004; Hebbeler et al., 2007) and the Pre-Elementary Education Longitudinal (PEELS) Study (Carlson et al., 2008; Markowitz et al., 2006) suggest that EI and ECSE are associated with positive developmental, social-emotional, language, and cognitive outcomes for children with disabilities.

The impact of EI and ECSE services on family outcomes, however, remains unclear. Based on a recent review of family outcome studies, Turnbull, Summers, Lee et al. (2007) reported that the large majority focus on how family outcomes vary as a function of individual (i.e., gender, type and severity of disability) or family (i.e., marital status, family income) characteristics. Among the studies that have examined the relationship between EI/ECSE services and family outcomes, findings are inconsistent. Based on data from the NEILS study, Bailey et al. (2006) and Hebbeler et al. (2007) reported that 90% to 96% of parents agreed or strongly agreed that EI/ESES services had enhanced their ability to meet their child's basic needs, help their child learn and develop, and work with professionals or advocate for services for their child. Conversely, Summers et al. (2007) found families with children birth to age 5 with a disability tended to believe they were not receiving enough family services to meet their needs. Examining the affect of EI services on family outcomes, Epley, Summers, and Turnbull (2008) found parent ratings of EI services significantly related to specific family outcomes (i.e., families know their rights and advocate effectively; understand their child's strengths, abilities, and needs; help their child develop and learn; have support systems; and access community services and activities) and overall family quality of life. These studies have not, however, examined how and to what extent EI/ECSE programs engage in family-centered practice or its effects on child and family outcomes. Consequently, research comparing conceptualizations and implementation of family-centered service delivery and its effect on child and family outcomes is warranted. Specifically, research should address how family-centered service delivery affects short-term family outcomes and the larger concept of family quality of life (Turnbull, Summers, Lee et al., 2007).

Limitations of This Review

Two aspects of our inclusionary criteria restricted the number of articles included in this review and should be considered limitations: the presence of an operational or constitutive definition and the inclusion of only peer-reviewed journal articles. Given our interest in how education and related fields conceptualize family-centered practice, only articles with explicit or relatively easily interpretable definitions were included. Although this criterion lessened the degree to which our own interpretations of family centeredness were included, more implicit understandings of family-centered practice were likely omitted. A second potential limitation is the inclusion of only peer-reviewed journal articles. Limiting conceptualizations of family centeredness to those published in peer-reviewed journals resulted in our excluding unpublished dissertations and scholarly presentations. Additionally, definitions of *family centeredness*, even those in perspective articles, primarily reflect the researchers' perspectives. A gap likely exists between the conceptualization and implementation of family-centered practice. As a result, conclusions drawn from this review are tentative.

CONCLUSION

We examined current definitions of *family-centered practice* using five key elements of Allen and Petr's (1996) benchmark definition: family as the unit of attention, family choice, family strengths, family–professional relationship, and individualized family services. Our review of articles published during the last decade indicates that though these elements remain central to conceptualizations of family centeredness, the emphasis on them has changed. Family-centered practice, once focused primarily on family as the unit of attention, is now largely associated with family choice. In fact, inclusion of family choice and a strengths-based perspective in definitions of *family centeredness* has increased whereas family as the unit of attention has declined.

It appears there is also an imbalance in the implementation of family centeredness and the provision of family services. Recommendations and strategies for family-centered practice overwhelmingly focused on relationship qualities and family–professional partnerships. The provision of services to families received much less attention. If we are to support young children with disabilities and their families, we must better prepare early childhood professionals for implementing family-centered practice, understand the relationship between family centeredness and outcomes for children with disabilities and their families, and assess not only child outcomes but also family outcomes.

REFERENCES

Allen, R. I., & Petr, C. G. (1996). Toward developing standards and measurements for family-centered practice in family support programs. In G. H. S. Singer, L. E. Powers, & A. L. Olson (Eds.), *Redefining family support* (pp. 57–84). Baltimore: Paul H. Brookes Publishing Co.

Bailey, D., Scarborough, A., Hebbeler, K., Spiker, D., & Mallik, S. (2004). *National early intervention longitudinal study: Family outcomes at the end of early intervention*. Menlo Park, CA: SRI International.

Bailey, D., Scarborough, A., Hebbeler, K., Spiker, D., & Mallik, S. (2006). *National early intervention longitudinal study: Family outcomes at the end of early intervention*. Menlo Park, CA: SRI International.

Bailey, D. B. (2001). Evaluating parent involvement and family support in early intervention and preschool programs. *Journal of Early Intervention, 24*(1), 1–14.

Bailey, D. B., McWilliams, R. A., Darkes, L. A., Hebbeler, K., Simeonsson, R. J., & Spiker, D., et al. (1998). Family outcomes in early intervention: A framework for program evaluation and efficacy research. *Exceptional Children, 64*(3), 313–329.

Blue-Banning, M., Summers, J. A., Frankland, H. C., Nelson, L. L., & Beegle, G. (2004). Dimensions of family and professional partnerships: Construction guidelines for collaboration. *Exceptional Children, 70*(2), 167–184.

Bodner-Johnson, B. (2001). Parents as adult learners in family-centered early education. *American Annals of the Deaf, 146*(3), 263–269.

Bruder, M. B. (2000). Family-centered early intervention: Clarifying our values for the new millennium. *Topics in Early Childhood Special Education, 20*(2), 105–122.

Campbell, P. H., & Halbert, J. (2002). Between research and practice: Provider perspectives on early intervention. *Topics in Early Childhood Special Education, 22*(4), 213–226.

Carlson, E., Daley, T., Shimshak, A., Riley, J., Keller, B., Jenkins, F., et al. (2008). *Changes in the characteristics, services, and performance of preschoolers with disabilities from 2003–04 to 2004–05: Wave 2 overview report from the Pre-Elementary Education Longitudinal Study (PEELS)*. Rockville, MD: Westat. Retrieved November 12, 2008, from https://www.peels.org/reports.asp

Crais, E. R., Roy, V. P., & Free, K. (2006). Parents' and professionals' perceptions of the implementation of family-centered practices in child assessments. *American Journal of Speech-Language Pathology, 15*, 365–377.

Cress, C. J. (2004). Augmentative and alternative communication and language: Understanding and responding to parents' perspectives. *Topics in Language Disorders, 24*(1), 51–61.

Danaher, J., & Armijo, C. (2005). *Part C updates* (7th ed.). Chapel Hill, NC: Frank Porter Graham Child Development Institute, National Early Childhood Technical Assistance Center.

Dunst, C., Trivette, C., & Deal, A. (1988). *Enabling and empowering families: Principles and guidelines for practice*. Cambridge, MA: Brookline.

Dunst, C. J., & Bruder, M. B. (2002). Valued outcomes of service coordination, early intervention, and natural environments. *Exceptional Children, 68*(3), 361–375.

Education of All Handicapped Children Act, 20 U.S.C. §1400 *et seq.* (1986).

Epley, P. H., Summers, J. A., & Turnbull, A. (2008). *Outcomes of early intervention: Relationships between service adequacy, family outcomes, and family quality of life*. Manuscript submitted for publication.

Erickson, K. A., Hatton, D., Roy, V., Fox, D., & Renne, D. (2007). Literacy in early intervention for children with visual impairments: Insights from individual cases. *Journal of Visual Impairment and Blindness*, *101*(2), 80–95.

Farmer, J. E., Clark, M. J., & Marien, W. E. (2003). Building systems of care for children with chronic health conditions. *Rehabilitation Psychology*, *48*(4), 242–249.

Fox, L., Dunlap, G., & Cushing, L. (2002). Early intervention, positive behavior support, and transition to school. *Journal of Emotional and Behavioral Disorders*, *10*(3), 149–157.

Friend, A. C., Summers, J. A., & Turnbull, A. P. (in press). Impacts of family support in early childhood intervention research. *Education and Training in Developmental Disabilities*, *44*(4), 453–470.

Gallagher, P. A., Rhodes, C. A., & Darling, S. M. (2004). Parents as professionals in early intervention: A parent educator model. *Topics in Early Childhood Special Education*, *24*(1), 5–13.

Grandlund, M., & Bjorck-Akesson, E. (2000). Integrating training in family-centered practices in context: Implications for implementing change activities. *Infants and Young Children*, *12*(3), 46–60.

Guillett, S. E. (2002). Preparing student nurses to provide home care for children with disabilities: A strengths-based approach. *Home Health Care Management and Practice*, *15*(1), 47–58.

Hamilton, M. E., Roach, M. A., & Riley, D. A. (2003). Moving toward family-centered early care and education: The past, the present, and a glimpse of the future. *Early Childhood Education Journal*, *30*(4), 225–232.

Hebbeler, K., Spiker, D., Bailey, D., Scarborough, A., Mallik, S., & Simeonsson, R., et al. (2007). *Early intervention for infants and toddlers with disabilities and their families: Participants, services, and outcomes* (SRI Project 11247). Menlo Park, CA: SRI International.

Herman, B. (2007). CAPTA and early childhood intervention: Policy and the role of parents. *Children and Schools*, *29*(1), 17–24.

King, G. A., Rosenbaum, P. L., & King, S. M. (1997). Evaluating family-centered service using a measure of parents' perceptions. *Child: Care, Health and Development*, *23*(1), 47–62.

Koller, D. F., Nicholas, D. B., Goldie, R. S., Gearing, R., & Selkirk, E. K. (2006). When family-centered care is challenged by infectious disease: Pediatric health care delivery during the SARS outbreaks. *Qualitative Health Research*, *16*(1), 47–60.

Larsson, M. (1999). Organising habilitation services: Team structures and family participation. *Child: Care, Health and Development*, *26*(6), 501–514.

Lea, D. (2006). "You don't know me like that": Patterns of disconnect between adolescent mothers of children with disabilities and their early interventionists. *Journal of Early Intervention*, *28*(4), 264–282.

Mahoney, G., & Bella, J. M. (1998). An examination of the effects of family-centered early intervention on child and family outcomes. *Topics in Early Childhood Special Education*, *18*(2), 83–94.

Mahoney, G., Kaiser, A., Girolametto, L., MacDonald, J., Robinson, C., & Safford, P., et al. (1999). Parent education in early intervention: A call for renewed focus. *Topics in Early Childhood Special Education*, *19*(3), 131–140.

Mandell, C. J., & Murray, M. M. (2005). Innovative family-centered practices in personnel preparation. *Teacher Education and Special Education, 28*(1), 74–77.

Markowitz, J., Carlson, E., Frey, W., Riley, J., Shimshak, A., & Heinzen, H., et al. (2006). *Preshoolers' characteristics, services, and results: Wave 1 Overview report from the Pre-Elementary Education Longitudinal Study (PEELS).* Rockville, MD: Westat. Retrieved November 12, 2008, from https://www.peels.org/reports.asp

McCormick, K. M., Vail, C., & Gallagher, P. A. (2002). Higher education consortia for early intervention: A survey of state efforts. *Teacher Education and Special Education, 25*(3), 298–308.

McWilliam, R. A., Snyder, P., Harbin, G. L., Porter, P., & Munn, D. (2000). Professionals' and families' perceptions of family-centered practices in infant-toddler services. *Early Education and Development, 11*(4), 519–538.

McWilliam, R. A., & Strain, P. S. (1993). Service delivery models: DEC recommended practices. In S. Sandall, M. E. McLean, & B. J. Smith (Eds.), *DEC recommended practices in early intervention/early childhood special education* (pp. 40–50). Longmont, CO: Sopris West. (ERIC Document Reproduction Service No. ED370258)

McWilliam, R. A., Tocci, L., & Harbin, G. L. (1998). Family-centered services: Service providers discourse and behavior. *Topics in Early Childhood Special Education, 18*(4), 206–221.

Murray, M., & Curran, E. (2008). Learning together with parents of children with disabilities: Bringing parent-professional partnership education to a new level. *Teacher Education and Special Education, 31*(1), 59–63.

Murray, M., & Mandell, C. (2004). Evaluation of a family-centered early childhood special education preservice model by program graduates. *Topics in Early Childhood Special Education, 24*(4), 238–249.

Murray, M. M., & Mandell, C. J. (2004). Evaluation of a family-centered early childhood special education preservice model by program graduates. *Topics in Early Childhood Special Education, 24*(4), 238–249.

Murray, M. M., & Mandell, C. J. (2006). On-the-job practices of early childhood special education providers trained in family-centered practices. *Journal of Early Intervention, 28*(2), 125–138.

National Early Childhood Technical Assistance Center. (2004). *IDEA Part C Early Intervention Services.* Retrieved September 27, 2007, from http://www.ideadata.org/arc_toc7.asp#partcEIS

Nelson, L. L., Summers, J. A., & Turnbull, A. P. (2004). Boundaries in family-professional partnerships: Implications for special education. *Remedial and Special Educators, 25*(3), 153–165.

Odom, S. L., & McLean, M. E. (1993). *DEC recommended practices: Indicators of quality in programs for infants and young children with special needs and their families.* DEC Task Force on Recommended Practices: Council for Exceptional Children.

Parette, H. P., & Brotherson, M. J. (2004). Family-centered and culturally responsive assistive technology decision making. *Infants and Young Children, 17*(4), 355–367.

Pretti-Frontczak, K., Giallourakis, A., Janas, D., & Hayes, A. (2002). Using a family-centered preservice curriculum to prepare early intervention and early childhood special education personnel. *Teacher Education and Special Education, 25*(3), 291–297.

Rao, S. (2000). Perspectives of an African American mother on parent-professional relationships in special education. *Mental Retardation, 38*(6), 475–488.

Ridgley, R., & Hallam, R. (2006). Examining the IFSPs of rural, low-income families: Are they reflective of family concerns? *Journal of Research in Childhood Education, 21*(2), 149–162.

Shelton, T. L., Jeppson, E. S., & Johnson, B. H. (1989). *Family-centered care for children with special health care needs* (2nd ed.). Washington, DC: Association for the Care of Children's Health.

Soodak, L. C., & Erwin, E. J. (2000). Valued member or tolerated participant: Parents' experiences in inclusive early childhood settings. *Journal of the Association for Persons with Severe Handicaps, 25*(1), 29–41.

Starble, A., Hutchins, T., Favro, M. A., Prelock, P., & Bitner, B. (2005). Family-centered intervention and satisfaction with AAC device training. *Communication Disorders Quarterly, 27*(1), 47–54.

Summers, J. A., Marquis, J., Mannan, H., Turnbull, A. P., Fleming, K., Poston, D. J., et al. (2007). Relationship of perceived adequacy of services, family-professional partnerships, and family quality of life in early childhood service programs. *International Journal of Developmental, Disability, and Education, 54*(3), 319–338.

Trivette, C. M., & Dunst, C. J. (2004). Evaluating family-based practices: Parenting experiences scale. *Young Exceptional Children, 7*(3), 12–19.

Trivette, C. M., & Dunst, C. J. (2005). DEC recommended practices: Family-based practices. In S. Sandall, M. L. Hemmeter, B. J. Smith, & M. E. McLean (Eds.), *DEC recommended practices: A comprehensive guide for practical application in early intervention/early childhood special education* (pp. 107–126). Longmont, CO: Sopris West.

Truesdale-Kennedy, M., McConkey, R., Ferguson, P., & Roberts, P. (2006). An evaluation of a family-centred support service for children with a significant learning disability. *Child Care in Practice, 12*(4), 377–390.

Turnbull, A. P., Summers, J. A., & Brotherson, M. J. (1984). *Working with families with disabled members: A family systems approach*. Lawrence: University of Kansas Affiliated Facility.

Turnbull, A. P., Summers, J. A., Lee, S. H., & Kyzar, K. (2007). Conceptualization and measurement of family outcomes associated with families of individuals with intellectual disabilities. *Mental Retardation and Developmental Disabilities, 13*, 346–356.

Turnbull, A. P., Summers, J. A., Turnbull, R., Brotherson, M. J., Winton, P., Roberts, R., et al. (2007). Family supports and services in early intervention: A bold vision. *Journal of Early Intervention, 29*(3), 187–206.

Vincent, L. J., & Beckett, J. A. (1993). Family participation: DEC recommended practices. In S. Sandall, M. E. McLean, & B. J. Smith (Eds.), *DEC recommended practices in early intervention/early childhood special education* (pp. 19–29). Longmont, CO: Sopris West. (ERIC Document Reproduction Service No. ED370256)

Winton, P., & Bailey, D. (1997). Family-centered care: The revolution continues. *The Exceptional Parent, 27*(2), 16–20.

Caregivers' Perceptions of a Consumer-Directed Care Program for Adults With Developmental Disabilities

LINDA VINTON

College of Social Work, Florida State University, Tallahassee, Florida

This article examines results from a consumer and caregiver-directed care pilot program for families with adults with developmental disabilities. Surveys were administered to 50 caregivers and three project coordinators, and focus groups were conducted with 44 individuals, including caregivers, consumers, and support coordinators. Significant pre- to posttest changes were seen in terms of caregivers' perceptions of choice, goodness-of-fit of services to needs, and satisfaction with the program. Analysis of focus group discussions yielded three major themes: trust, flexibility, and relief. Although support and program coordinators had some concerns that the program was more caregiver than consumer oriented at times, overall, the program was viewed positively.

The National Alliance for Caregiving (2009) defines *caregivers of adults* as persons who provide "unpaid care to a relative or friend 18 years or older to help them take care of themselves." *Unpaid care* is defined as "help with personal needs or household chores. It might be managing a person's finances, arranging for outside services, or visiting regularly" (p. 2). It has been estimated that more than 75% of adults with developmental disabilities

This project was funded by the Florida Department of Children and Families. The author would like to acknowledge Dr. Robin Perry for contributions regarding the cost analyses for the project, René Schwallie who assisted with coding focus group data, and Dr. Bruce Thyer for his comments. An earlier analysis of cost and satisfaction data was presented by the author and Dr. Robin Perry at the Annual Meeting of the Southeast Evaluation Association in Tallahassee, Florida, in January 2003.

live at home with at least one family member (Fujiura, 1998). Developmental disabilities programs that allow for consumer or surrogate direction, such as by a family caregiver, have become increasingly popular. Furthermore, it has been reported that 80% of consumer-directed programs in the United States allow consumers to hire family members to provide care (Doty & Flanagan, 2002). Utilization of the term *consumers* in human services departs from notions of *patients, clients*, and even *care receivers*, in that consumers are viewed as having a strong desire for self-determination and to be most knowledgeable in terms of what types and amounts of services are needed (Friedman, 2007).

Consumer-directed programs have earlier roots in the Veteran's Administration Housebound and Aid and Attendance Allowance Program (Cameron, 1993), as well as the independent living movement (DeJong, Batavia, & McKnew, 1992). Robert Wood Johnson Foundation and other government-sponsored consumer-directed long-term care models have also subsequently been developed that are aimed not only at persons with disabilities, but also at family members in particular (Ansello & Eustis, 1992; Benjamin & Matthias, 2000; Moseley, 1999; Velgouse & Dize, 2000). Community integration of persons with disabilities was the focus of the U.S. Supreme Court's 1999 decision in *Olmstead v L.C.* (527 U.S. 581). The Court affirmed that integration was an obligation of public programs under the Americans with Disabilities Act (ADA) Title II (28 CFR 35, 1991). In line with the decision, the Centers for Medicare and Medicaid Services Real Choice Initiative and the New Freedom Commission (2003) supported community-based long-term services with an emphasis on individualized care plans (Powers, Sowers, & Singer, 2006).

Choice making and self-determination go hand in hand. Choice involves "the opportunity to make an uncoerced selection from two or more alternative(s)" (Bannerman, Sheldon, Sherman, & Harchik, 1991, p. 80). Defined as "a combination of skills, knowledge, and beliefs that enable a person to engage in goal-directed, self-regulated, autonomous behavior" (Field, Martin, Miller, Ward, & Wehmeyer, 1998, p. 2), self-determination is undergirded by values that have influenced the design of consumer-directed support programs. Belief in the rights of all people to decide or make choices for themselves is thus seen as an individual rights issue in the field of disability services (Guess, Benson, & Siegel-Causey, 1985; Shevin & Klein, 1984; Wehmeyer, 1998). A major goal of consumer-directed support programs is to shift more authority and responsibility for the direction or nature of supports to consumers and/or their representatives (Caldwell, 2007; Powers et al., 2006). Other objectives of consumer-driven care models include normalization, support employment, community housing options, and positive behavior support that encourage treatment of people with dignity and respect (Wood, Fowler, Uphold, & Test, 2005).

Promoting personal autonomy in making choices about one's own care may be limited by cognitive disabilities, and case managers have expressed concern regarding unbounded autonomy in the face of safety issues (Micco, Hamilton, Martin, & McEwan, 1995; Scala, Mayberry, & Kunkel, 1996). Reflective of such concerns, consumer-directed programs tend to be bounded (e.g., criteria are established for decision makers and decision making) or allow surrogates such as family members, guardians, or other types of caregivers to make decisions, while encouraging collaboration between consumers and trusted others (Powers et al., 2006).

Although researchers have examined program costs and rates of institutionalization in the past, the literature on perceptions of family caregivers is growing, along with the number of consumer-directed family support programs that serve families with adult relatives with developmental disabilities (National Council on Disability, 2004; Rizzolo, Hemp, & Braddock, 2006). Consumer-directed care programs have been implemented with different populations across home- and community-based settings. They range from consumers or surrogates having minimal control (e.g., having a role at care plan meetings) to maximum control over the type and amount of services, as well as who provides the service and how much the provider is paid (Velgouse & Dize, 2000). To assess awareness and interest by state administrators in consumer-directed care projects, the National Institute on Disability and Rehabilitation Research awarded a grant to the National Council on Aging to conduct two surveys (Valgouse & Dize, 2000). The second survey in 1999 found that state administrators' awareness of consumer direction and cash and counseling programs had increased since the first survey in 1996.

The nature of consumer-directed programs was explored in the National Council on Aging surveys. Among the developmental disabilities and Medicaid programs, nonagency personnel (e.g., friends, neighbors, family members other than spouses and responsible parent) were the most frequent providers of service as reported by more than 75% of these respondents. Reimbursement methods also showed a shift toward consumer control; although 75% of the programs in the 1996 survey used direct payment to providers, this had dropped to half of the programs in 1999. The proportion of programs that offered cash payments to consumers or surrogates was not found to change (about 35%); rather, the use of fiscal intermediaries increased.

California's In-Home Support Services program is directed at consumers who live in their own homes, have incomes within the Supplemental Security Income guidelines, and are aged, disabled, or blind (Benjamin & Matthias, 2000). The program turns over the responsibilities for finding, hiring, training, and monitoring caregivers to consumers. Workers can include family members or others selected by the client and are paid directly by the state once their hours are certified by the client. An hourly rate (usually minimum wage) has been established by the state for these purposes. It has been reported that more than 40% of the providers of services within this program are relatives of the clients and approximately 25% are friends or acquaintances.

One of the larger consumer-directed care projects, the Cash and Counseling Demonstration and Evaluation program, has been implemented in three states. These programs allow adult consumers or their surrogates, usually family members, to directly purchase services and pay for other resources needed by consumers, rather than use vendor payments or vouchers to pay for care. With guidance from focus groups, researchers evaluated the Cash and Counseling Demonstration program using a telephone survey that asked about frequency and satisfaction with services and perceptions regarding the cash option (Simon-Rusinowitz, Mahoney, Loughlin, & Sadler, 2005; Simon-Rusinowitz et al., 2001). A total of 378 persons (100 consumers and 278 surrogates) responded, yielding a 53% response rate. Although 79% of the respondents were satisfied with current services (e.g., case manager, transportation, adult day training), results indicated that 45% of the consumers/surrogates said that they would like to have greater say in the selection of services, and 35% wanted greater control over when services were received.

In other evaluations of the Cash and Counseling Demonstration program, family caregivers of program participants were compared to a randomly selected comparison group (Foster, Brown, Phillips, & Carlson, 2005a, 2005b, 2005c). Program caregivers were less likely to have high levels of physical and financial strain and less likely to report negative impacts of giving care on their social lives, jobs, and privacy. They reported greater life satisfaction and satisfaction with services than the comparison group.

In an evaluation of the Illinois Home Based Support Services Program, Caldwell (2006) surveyed 209 primary family caregivers of adults with developmental disabilities enrolled in the program and 85 families on a waitlist. Although respondents represented a relatively small percentage of the recruitment sample (30.2% and 15.3%, respectively), the use of waitlisted families as controls allowed the researcher to compare the impact of having supports. Caregivers participating in the program were found to engage in more social activities and to have greater leisure satisfaction than caregivers on the waitlist. It was also reported that among lower income families, caregiver participants had better mental health and greater access to health care than nonparticipants.

When repeated measures were used over time to examine unmet needs, service satisfaction, community participation, and caregiving burden for a random sample participating in the Illinois Home Based Support Services Program, Caldwell and Heller (2007) found that unmet needs decreased, service satisfaction increased, and community participation increased between baseline and 4 years after entering the program. No significant differences were found between the intermediate time and

5 years later (note that only 38 of the original 135 families returned surveys). Although no change was seen in caregiver burden between baseline and 4 years later, caregiver burden decreased significantly during the subsequent 5-year period.

Although the range of control over the type and amount of services has varied in terms of consumer-directed programs, the literature has primarily focused on quantitative evaluations of programs where minimal to moderate control could be exercised (e.g., who could be paid to provide help was restricted or rates for services were established by a state office). In this study, consumers and caregivers were given maximum control (e.g., not restricted to Medicaid-approved providers or certain provider rates or monthly care plan amounts) with the exception of using a fiduciary, and a qualitative evaluation was added. In addition to being able to more thoroughly evaluate caregivers' perceptions of and satisfaction with the program, the extent to which they chose to exert maximum control (e.g., provide care within the family only or not hire a support coordinator) could also be examined.

METHOD

The Program

The current study looked at the perceptions of caregivers or consumer representatives who took part in a state-funded consumer and caregiver-directed pilot program that was implemented for a fixed time (originally 2 years but scaled back to just over a year) in three geographic areas of one southeastern state. All of the participants in the program had previous experience with a Home and Community-Based Services (HCBS) Medicaid Waiver model whereby developmental services agencies provided case management and would pay fixed amounts to Medicaid-approved providers from state-maintained lists of providers.

The consumer and caregiver-directed care program was supported with state funds, along with monies from a developmental disabilities council. Interest in a state only, versus foundation-funded (e.g., Robert Wood Johnson) or combination federal-state funded program, was the result of family members and advocates for persons with disabilities making requests to state legislators for a program that would better serve the needs of consumers. In particular, there was concern over reports of maltreatment and malfeasance by Medicaid providers. Family members believed they could provide better care themselves or hire non-Medicaid providers that would be more knowledgeable and caring.

Staff from the state's developmental disabilities services office worked with local coalitions of family members of persons with developmental disabilities, consumers, service providers, and other interested persons in developing the program. Aspects of the program that distinguished it from other state-funded developmental services included (1) greater choice over type and amount of services, (2) control of funds (one area used zero-based budgeting and the others used previous plans to estimate costs), (3) choice over hiring providers (including non-Medicaid providers such as family members), and (4) flexible purchasing guidelines. Caregivers or consumers coordinated services or hired a support coordinator. Only a small number of consumers acted as their own representatives, but most consumers were able to communicate choices. Caregivers (referred to as consumer representatives by the program) were offered limited-service or full-service fiscal intermediary assistance with such things as employment taxes, labor laws, and managing funds. The fiduciary agency was located outside the state and had experience with consumer-directed programs.

Types of services that adults with developmental disabilities commonly used before and after participating in the consumer- and family-directed care program were personal care, nursing/medical, respite, and homemaker/chore services. In terms of resources, care plans often reflected the need for consumable medical supplies, transportation, and home modifications and/or equipment. Care plans also included social companionship, day activities, training, and respite services for caregivers.

The cost of monthly care plans had to be approved by the program director who worked through the State office for persons with disabilities. The amount of each plan was not fixed but rather started either at $0 or with the monthly cost of plans prior to joining the program. As with the cash and carry programs, it was expected that costs would not increase because money-saving strategies could be employed such as negotiating rates or cutting back on services that family members could provide, including case management (Kapp, 1996; Simon-Rusinowitz et al., 2001).

Consumers and Caregivers

Consumers were clients of a state developmental disabilities services program who were referred by staff to the consumer and family-directed care pilot program. To be eligible, consumers had to be at least age 18 years; have a developmental disability that included mental retardation, autism, cerebral palsy, spina bifida, or Prader-Willi syndrome; reside in the community; and be a resident of three targeted geographic areas. The vast majority of consumers lived with a family caregiver who acted as their representative. Representatives provided care and arranged for care of consumers, but some preferred to hire a support coordinator for assistance with case management. Again, caregiver representatives had a choice of who to hire, but some already had a support coordinator prior to the program. Each consumer had one primary caregiver for the purposes of the study, usually a parent or a sibling.

Measures

The program was conducted in three geographic areas. Each area had a project coordinator. At the conclusion of the program, project coordinators were interviewed and completed a brief survey. Items they were asked about included the pros and cons of the program, issues that came to their attention throughout the program, perceptions of changes to consumers' quality of life as the result of the program, and beliefs about consumer direction in general.

Pre- and posttest surveys were developed for caregivers that examined perception of choice, activities choice, goodness of fit of services to consumer's needs, and satisfaction with services and the program. Questions were derived from two stated goals of the program: (1) to get the services and support that best meet the needs of individuals and their families and (2) to give individuals and their families more choice about what services they get, who provides them, and how often. Items were discussed and approved by an external evaluator, program administrators, and a consultant researcher with expertise in working with adults with developmental disabilities. Pretests were administered at baseline or prior to participating in the program, and posttests were administered 6 months after starting on the program. The program was scheduled to last for a second year, and some 12-month follow-up surveys were completed; however, recruitment was staggered and the program ended earlier than planned, so there were too few participants whose pretest, posttest, and follow-up surveys could be matched and analyzed.

Perception of choice

Participants were asked the extent to which they agreed that they had choice over (1) what services were provided, (2) who performed services, (3) how the services were provided, (4) how much service was provided, (5) how to spend money that paid for services, and (6) hiring a support coordinator. A Likert-type scale was used for responses (1 = *strongly agree*, 2 = *agree*, 3 = *disagree*, 4 = *strongly disagree*).

Activities choice

The Activities Choice Survey asked caregivers if caregivers wanted to make a change in their daily activities or to do more or less of certain activities such as visiting with family, friends, or participate in recreational and social activities.

Fit of services to needs

Two items addressed goodness of fit on the Satisfaction Survey. The first asked participants to what extent they agreed that the type of services received all matched the needs of the consumer, and the second inquired if the amount of service was sufficient to meet the consumer's needs. Both used Likert-type response categories (1 = *strongly agree*, 2 = *agree*, 3 = *disagree*, 4 = *strongly disagree*).

Satisfaction

The Satisfaction Survey asked if services could be secured for consumers in a timely manner and whether caregivers were satisfied with the quality of services. Another item asked if caregivers were satisfied with the number of times their requests for services or resources were honored by the program and if they felt comfortable asking program staff questions about the program. Finally, caregivers were asked if they believed that services received contributed positively to the consumer's quality of life. Again, Likert-type response categories were used (1 = *strongly agree*, 2 = *agree*, 3 = *disagree*, 4 = *strongly disagree*).

Focus Groups

In addition to the collection of survey data, the author conducted seven 90-minute focus groups with family caregivers, consumers, service providers, and support coordinators. Extensive notes were taken by the author that followed the questions in a protocol script (discussion guide) approved by a Human Subjects Committee, but comments were not recorded. Program participants (consumers, caregivers, other representatives, support coordinators, and service providers) were invited to attend by the program administrator. Focus groups were held in each area where the program had been operating for at least 6 months. Krueger (1994) stated that focus groups bring together individuals with a common interest (in this case, care for adults with developmental disabilities) who can share information about a specific issue (consumer/caregiver-directed care). The atmosphere of focus groups allows for persons to express their perceptions without having to reach consensus. This is important in terms of caregivers who may feel their voices have been lacking when it comes to developmental disabilities program development and who have different points of view. A discussion guide was prepared in advance with questions to guide discussion (Greenbaum, 2000). Questions were asked about caregivers' experience with care providers, how the program affected caregivers' and consumers' lives, and how the program compared to the traditional system of service.

Data Analysis

For the purposes of the current study, Krueger's (1994) framework was used for the analysis of focus group data. The analysis continuum consists of raw data, descriptive statements, and interpretation. The steps are to examine frequency, specificity, emotions, and extensiveness of words, and then to develop "big ideas" or themes. Data are reread accordingly, and preliminary notes are taken that are used to develop a beginning outline or system for classifying comments. These are the broad "regularities" that become themes (Marshall & Rossman, 1999). The author and a research assistant independently reviewed the data using this process and developed and applied a coding system. In those cases where statements were coded differently, an alternating strategy was employed (first rater's coding selected, then second rater's, etc.).

Pretest and 6-month posttest survey responses were analyzed using matched pair *t* tests and the Bonferonni correction to guard against test-wise error. Although the program ran for more than 12 months and involved 143 consumers, there were too few 12-month posttests that could be matched to pretests and 6-month posttests for a meaningful analysis.

RESULTS

Demographics

Slightly more than half of the consumers were male, and the age range was 18 to 57 ($M = 28.4$) (see Table 1). Three fifths of the consumers were White; and among the minority participants, most were African American. Three fourths of the consumers lived with their parents, and only rarely did a consumer live alone. Primary diagnoses tended most often to be mild, moderate, severe, or profound mental retardation (78%), followed by multiple diagnoses (10%), cerebral palsy (8%), spina bifida (2%), and autism (2%). On a scale of 1 (*limited*) to 5 (*extensive*), approximately one half had needs deemed to be intensive or extensive.

Demographics of caregivers were not collected, with the exception of those who attended focus groups. Although each of the 50 consumers either represented himself or herself or had a representative of record, consumers tended to have more than one caregiver; thus, the total number of caregivers was difficult to establish. Roughly three fourths of the representatives of record were parents of consumers and another 10% were other relatives. The seven focus groups were attended by 44 persons: 24 family caregivers (parents and siblings of consumers), 3 parent caregivers not serving as the primary representative, 2 nonfamily caregivers, 9 consumers, 4 service providers; and 2 support coordinators. Of the 38 caregivers and consumers, 29 were female and 9 were male, and 25 were White, 12 African American, and 1 Asian American.

Activities Choice

At pretest, consumers' daily activities included part-time (9%) or full-time paid work (13%), school (25%) or day program (34%), unpaid work (6%),

TABLE 1 Consumer (Adult With Developmental Disability) Demographics ($N = 50$)

	%
Gender	
Male	58
Female	42
Race/ethnicity	
White	60
African American	30
Other	6
Asian American	2
Indian/Alaska Native	2
Age (Range 18–57)	
18–21	26
22–29	31
30–44	41
45+	2
Living arrangement	
With parents	76
With friend/Nonparent relative	11
Alone	7
Nonfamily Home with supervision	6
Primary diagnosis	
Mild retardation	15
Moderate retardation	23
Severe retardation	19
Profound retardation	21
Cerebral palsy	8
Spina bifida	2
Autism	2
Multiple	10
Level of need	
Limited	20
Minimal	6
Moderate	25
Intensive	10
Extensive	39

or activities at home only (13%). Thirty-five percent of the caregivers indicated that consumers wanted a change in their daily activities. At posttest, there was virtually no change, and 34% said a daily activities change was desired. Although five consumers moved to more independent or paid activities during this time, four moved to less independent or unpaid activities.

At pretest, almost all (96%) of the consumers had daily or weekly contact with family members, but 17% of the caregivers reported consumers wanted more contact with family. At posttest, the percentage dropped slightly to 13% that indicated consumers wanted more contact with family. At pretest, 66% of consumers saw their friends daily or weekly, and 42% of the caregivers said more contact was desired. At posttest, this percentage decreased to 23%. At pretest, 60% of the consumers were involved in fun or social activities on a daily or weekly basis, and a majority (57%) of caregivers reported that these activities were desired more often. At posttest, only 29% said that consumers wanted more fun and social activities.

Perceptions of Choice, Goodness of Fit of Services to Needs, and Program Satisfaction

For all items, there were significant increases from pre- to posttest (see Table 2). Perceptions at pretest as to choices regarding support coordination, who performed services, how funds were spent, what services were provided, how services were provided, and how much service was provided yielded mean ratings between 2.51 (choice over support coordinator) and 3.37 (choice over spending), where a rating of 1 indicated a strong positive perception and 4 indicated a strong negative perception. Compared to pretest, posttest mean ratings of perceptions of choice items were less variable and ranged from 1.36 to 1.65.

Similar results were seen for perceptions of the goodness of fit of services to consumers' needs. Mean ratings of 2.69 (services matched needs) and 2.93 (amount of services were sufficient) at pretest, compared to 1.40 and 1.65, respectively, at posttest.

Some of the lowest (most positive) ratings at pretest were found for program satisfaction items. Means ranged from 2.11 and 2.14 for the two

TABLE 2 Perceptions of Choice, Goodness of Fit, and Satisfaction With Program

	Pretest		Posttest				95% CI		
Item	*M*	*SD*	*M*	*SD*	*t*(49)	*p*	LL	UL	Cohen's *d*
Perceptions of Choice									
Who performed services	2.86	.948	1.36	.598	9.55	.000	1.18	1.82	0.69
Spending	3.37	.727	1.57	.764	11.86	.000	1.49	2.10	0.77
What services	2.76	.894	1.38	.490	9.88	.000	1.10	1.67	0.69
How services provided	3.04	.763	1.47	.616	10.78	.000	1.28	1.87	0.75
How much service	3.06	.836	1.65	.812	9.02	.000	1.10	1.73	0.65
Support coordinator[a]	2.51	.944	1.36	.609	6.15	.000	0.78	1.53	0.59
Perceptions of Goodness of Fit									
Matched needs	2.69	.748	1.40	.707	9.96	.000	1.03	1.56	0.66
Amount enough	2.93	.800	1.65	.766	8.31	.000	0.97	1.59	0.63
Perceptions of Satisfaction									
Timely manner	2.77	.928	1.52	.714	8.01	.000	0.94	1.56	0.60
Can ask staff	2.48	.937	1.39	.577	7.49	.000	0.79	1.38	0.57
Can ask coordinators[a]	2.11	.843	1.46	.650	3.92	.000	0.31	0.98	0.40
Coordinator help[a]	2.14	.787	1.62	.758	2.99	.005	0.17	0.86	0.32
Quality of life	2.41	.956	1.29	.677	6.64	.000	0.78	1.46	0.56
Quality of services	2.81	.816	1.31	.624	9.89	.000	1.20	1.81	0.72
Requests granted	2.76	.860	1.41	.670	8.68	.000	1.03	1.65	0.66

Note: CI = confidence interval; LL = lower limit; UL = upper limit.
[a]$N = 37$ for support coordinator items.

items related to support coordination (comfortable asking the support coordinator questions and able to get help from the support coordinator) to 2.81 (satisfaction with quality of services). At posttest program satisfaction mean ratings ranged from 1.29 (satisfaction with quality of services) to 1.62 (able to get help from the support coordinator).

Project Coordinators' Responses

Three project coordinators administered the consumer and caregiver-directed care program in different geographic areas. Although they were surveyed about individual consumers, in-person interviews yielded responses to open-ended questions about the program's strengths and weaknesses (see Table 3) and perceptions of consumer-directed care in general. With respect to their thoughts about consumer-directed programs, the coordinators noted

TABLE 3 Project Coordinators' Perceptions of Strengths and Weaknesses of the Program ($N=3$)

Strengths	Weaknesses
Participants liked the freedom or leeway in devising care plans.	Some amounts of service were so small that it is unlikely that the service increased quality of life.
More caring workers were hired.	Some representatives could have done better in providing needed care.
Families could be paid for care, and this helped them financially and emotionally.	A consumer became involved with Adult Protective Services and had to come off the project.
Consumers could get as much help as they actually needed.	Some family members were paid much higher hourly rates than other family members and some were not paid at all.
Allowing money for adult briefs	Much variation and unreasonable rates paid to workers.
Family care costs less than nonfamily care.	Families insisted on providing most of the care, but consumers needed other services.
Quality of care is higher if provided by a family member.	Families were not as accountable as service providers–they do not keep case notes, etc.
Family members now feel their care is worth something.	Representatives overlooked recreational and social activities that consumers wanted.
Families can enjoy a better standard of living when paid for caregiving.	Some had difficulty putting together care plans and thinking in new ways or "outside the box."
Families can be there 24 hours a day 7 days a week if needed.	Finding reliable nonfamily workers could be difficult.
Positive behavioral changes in consumers were seen because of type and quality of care provided.	The project manual was not useful for many (some did not need it, some did not read it, and some had trouble understanding it).
Consumers were able to get therapies and equipment such as communication devices and lifts that were not accessible before or took years to get.	Some services were not covered, and this angered participants.
For consumers in more remote areas it was difficult to get workers – the project helped to pay the workers enough so they would come long distances to work.	The program had to be explained over and over to service or resource providers.
Dental needs got met.	
Participants got more "bang for the buck."	

that choice models were preferred by family members but that financial issues could be confusing and contentious. They believed that all consumers and family members needed fiscal assistance and access to comprehensive social work services. They also noted that uniform administration of programs should be a goal and that networking meetings and consumer governing boards should be a part of every consumer-directed care program.

Focus Group Responses

Trust

The first major theme identified was trust (having trust in providers). Most of the family caregivers, as well as two consumers, recounted negative experiences prior to enrolling in the consumer and caregiver-directed care program. They described instances when Medicaid-approved service providers had been incompetent, uncaring, unreliable, and had even been abusive to consumers. Under the program, they knew they could find someone who already knew the consumer, was familiar with his or her needs, or could be trained by the family caregiver. Caregivers expressed how important it was for workers to understand not only the limitations of consumers, but also to get to know the consumer (personality, habits, likes and dislikes). Examples of "trust" statements included:

- I can train and get people I know.
- Providers now are predictable.
- I can hire someone who is not familiar with group homes . . . and not burned out.
- The people that now work with my son know about autism, are trained, and understand how sensory stimulation works.
- Nobody loves our children like we do.
- The worker used to call my son by the wrong name.
- Now I can be there with a provider at first to see how they are doing with my child.

Flexibility

The second major theme identified was flexibility. Family caregivers stated that the program enabled them to more easily respond to situations that required resources or services. This gave them "peace of mind" knowing that they could change a care plan as needed and even request additional funds because the budgeting process was done for a period of time. They noted instances of illness, surgery, and an accident where consumers needed extensive care for a limited period of time. They also mentioned the importance of flexibility in regard to their own inability to provide care due to health problems, and how the program allowed them to move on to "Plan B" when needed. Examples of "flexibility" statements included:

- We cut out the supportive living coach and use the money for direct care now.
- We needed help in an emergency and that was possible with [the program].
- We won't have to have a different person doing the job we already are doing.
- We added some recreational things and it's nice that my child's brothers and sisters can do things with him now.
- We heard that others added things like exercise programs to their plans and that's a good idea.
- We can be more creative although we still have to justify [expenses].

Relief

The third major theme identified was relief. The consumer and family directed-care program was viewed by family caregivers as giving them more freedom to go to paid jobs, do recreational activities, spend time with other family members and friends, and to have respite from being a caregiver. When asked how the consumer and family directed-care program compared to the traditional system, participants were almost unanimous in their belief that the program was an improvement, and they were eager, almost desperate, for the program to continue past the pilot phase. Examples of "relief" statements included:

- It's just reassuring to know you can get who you want to take care of your child.
- [The program] allows me to work and I'll need the Social Security benefits when I retire.
- We may be able to get out of debt in a year or so.
- We can have some time off since we can pay others to do certain services like transportation.
- I couldn't be here today if it weren't for the project because now I can get and pay for a sitter on short notice.
- I can get out.
- I went through many jobs in many years because I had to take off to deal with crises; now I can work.

DISCUSSION

The shortened timeframe and inability to use consumers' surveys have already been mentioned as limitations of the current study. In addition, the pretest–posttest design would have been strengthened by using a comparison group (Shadish, Cook, & Campbell, 2002), although it can be noted that effect sizes were between medium and large. It is common in conducting program evaluations to attempt to overcome weaknesses in quasi-experimental designs by using a multimethod, multiple perspective approach (Patton, 2002). This was attempted, as quantitative and qualitative data were collected from caregivers, project coordinators, and others in attendance at focus groups.

Services that better matched the needs of consumers were more frequently accessed through the consumer and caregiver-directed care program described herein, and family caregivers' perceptions of choice and satisfaction with activities and services significantly increased between start-up (pretest) and 6 months later (posttest). This was not surprising, given what we know from the literature, particularly the Illinois Home Based Support Services Program that surveyed family caregivers of adults with developmental disabilities and controls, and the Cash and Counseling Demonstration program that included elderly and nonelderly consumers.

Prior to the program, services were included in consumers' cost plans that were not utilized, resulting in funds being unexpended and needs being unmet. Focus group participants attributed this to the poor quality of Medicaid-approved providers. Caregivers were reluctant to hire persons they did not know and could not necessarily trust with their disabled family members. Through the consumer and caregiver-directed care program, most representatives paid family members and friends to provide services, thus caregivers came to associate trust, flexibility, and relief with the program. This is what the qualitative data yielded in this particular study, therefore adding information about why caregivers responded as they did at posttest.

The current study also looked beyond caregivers in terms of perspectives about the program. Although cash allowance programs tend to please caregivers in particular, the three project coordinators interviewed for the current study, along with the support coordinators and consumers who took part in focus groups, pointed to some problem areas in terms of programs that allow family members to coordinate, provide, and be paid for care of adults with developmental disabilities. On the one hand, when given choice and control over funds, caregivers tended to provide more of the care themselves or to pay other family members. Some caregivers in the current study stated that they were more familiar not only with their family member's wants and needs than agency workers but also with local resources and services. These families tended to network with and learn from other families and at the same time received emotional support from other caregivers who they considered to be "in the know."

On the other hand, it was noted that some parent caregivers took the "I know what's best" approach in terms of resources and activities for their adult children and were not open to the consumer's choices. Although the researcher attempted to survey consumers for the current study, it became a validity issue when caregivers filled out consumers' questionnaires. Nevertheless, in response to the item, "Would you like to change what you do during the day?" almost two thirds of the consumers (or their representatives) answered *yes*, and said they wanted to do things such as join an exercise class, clean houses, volunteer, go to school, or work. When caregivers were surveyed about daily activities though, 35% indicated that consumers wanted a change at pretest and 34% said the same at posttest. The percentage that reported consumers wanted more contact with friends decreased from pre- to posttest but was still relatively high (23%) at posttest. The same was true for desiring more fun or social activities (29% reported consumers wanted more of such activities at posttest).

Caregivers in the current study strongly favored a consumer-directed approach to care for adults with developmental disabilities. From what was said in the focus groups, it appeared the primary reason appeared to be protective. As family members who were responsible for vulnerable adults, they pointed to past experiences with poor caretakers and were highly motivated to find caring and competent caregivers for their loved ones. They also stated their own reasons for liking the program. They found it easier to line up services and resources when needed, rather than have to gain approval ahead of time by way of care plans, case managers, and state agencies.

When consumer and caregivers' interests do not match, however, it is not always clear how to respect client self-determination. Although the intent of consumer-directed care programs is obvious in the name, "clients" of such programs can be viewed more broadly to mean consumers and their surrogates or caregivers. It is a delicate balance to respect the rights of individual consumers and caregivers to make choices about care and how to spend funds allocated for care, and yet promote self-determination at the same time. Consumer-directed care programs should recognize this and have some mechanism in place to help promote consumers' choices.

REFERENCES

Ansello, E. F., & Eustis, N. N. (1992). A common stake? Investigating the emerging intersection of aging and disabilities. *Generations, 16*, 5–8.

Bannerman, D. J., Sheldon, J. B., Sherman, J. A., & Harchik, A. E. (1991). Balancing the right to habilitation with the right to personal liberties: The rights of people with developmental disabilities to eat too many doughnuts and take a nap. *Journal of Applied Behavior Analysis, 23*, 79–89.

Benjamin, A. E., & Matthias, R. E. (2000). Comparing consumer- and agency-directed models: California's in-home supportive services program. *Generations, 24*, 85–87.

Caldwell, J. (2006). Consumer-directed supports: Economic, health, and social outcomes for families. *Mental Retardation, 44*, 405–417.

Caldwell, J. (2007). Experiences of families with relatives with intellectual and developmental disabilities in a consumer-directed support program. *Disability & Society, 22*, 549–562.

Caldwell, J., & Heller, T. (2007). Longitudinal outcomes of a consumer-directed program supporting adults with developmental disabilities and their families. *Intellectual and Developmental Disabilities, 45*, 161–173.

Cameron, K. A. (1993). *International and domestic programs using "cash and counseling" strategies to pay for long-term care.* Washington, DC: United Seniors Health Cooperative.

DeJong, G., Batavia, A. E., & McKnew, L. (1992). The independent living model of personal assistance in national long-term care policy. *Generations, 16*, 89–95.

Doty, P., & Flanagan, S. (2002). *Highlights: Inventory of consumer-directed support programs* Washington, DC: U.S. Department of Health and Human Services, Aging and Long-Term Care Policy, Office of Disability. Retrieved from http://aspe.hhs.gov/daltcp/Reports/highlght.htm

Field, S., Martin, J., Miller, R., Ward, M., & Wehmeyer, M. (1998). *A practical guide to teaching self-determination*. Reston, VA: Council for Exceptional Children.

Foster, L., Brown, R., Phillips, B., & Carlson, B. L. (2005a). Easing the burden of caregiving: The impact of consumer direction on primary informal care in Arkansas. *The Gerontologist, 45*, 474–485.

Foster, L., Brown, R., Phillips, B., & Carlson, B. L. (2005b). *The effects of cash and counseling on the primary informal caregivers of children with developmental disabilities.* Washington, DC: U.S. Department of Health and Human Services, Aging and Long-Term Care Policy, Office of Disability, Office of the Assistant Secretary for Planning and Evaluation. Retrieved from http://www.cashandcounseling.org/resources/20060120-105320/ddkidpic.pdf

Foster, L., Brown, R., Phillips, B., & Carlson, B. L. (2005c). *How cash and counseling affects informal caregivers: Findings from Arkansas, Florida, and New Jersey.* Washington, DC: U.S. Department of Health and Human Services, Aging and Long-Term Care Policy, Office of Disability, Office of the Assistant Secretary for Planning and Evaluation. Retrieved from http://aspe.hhs.gov/daltcp/reports/ICaffectes.htm

Friedman, E. (2007). The new meaning of caring: Forces reshaping 21st century health care. In The National Center on Caregiving at Family Caregiver Alliance in Partnership with The American Society on Aging (Eds.), *Conference proceedings: Family caregiving: State of the art, Future trends* (pp. 4–10). Retrieved from http://www.caregiver.org/caregiver/jsp/content/pdfs/2007_asa_preconference_proceedingsII.pdf

Fujiura, G. T. (1998). Demography of family households. *American Journal on Mental Retardation, 103*, 225–235.

Greenbaum, T. (2000). *Moderating focus groups: A practical guide for group facilitation*. Thousand Oaks, CA: Sage.

Guess, D., Benson, H. A., & Siegal-Causey, E. (1985). Concepts and issues related to choice-making and autonomy among persons with severe disabilities. *Journal of the Association for Persons with Severe Handicaps, 10*, 79–86.

Kapp, M. (1996). Enhancing autonomy and choice in selecting and directing long-term care services. *Elder Law Journal*, *4*, 55–97.

Krueger, R. A. (1994). *Focus groups: A practical guide for applied research* (2nd ed.). Newbury Park, CA: Sage.

Marshall, C., & Rossman, G. B. (1999). *Designing qualitative research* (3rd ed.). Thousand Oaks, CA: Sage.

Micco, A., Hamilton, A. C. S., Martin, M. J., & McEwan, K. L. (1995). Case manager attitudes toward client-centered care. *Journal of Case Management*, *4*, 95–101.

Moseley, C. (1999). *Making self determination work*. Durham: University of New Hampshire, National Program Office on Self-Determination, Institute on Disability.

National Alliance for Caregiving in Collaboration with AARP. (2009). *Caregiving in the U.S.* Retrieved from http://assets.aarp.org/rgcenter/il/caregiving_09_fr.pdf

National Council on Disability. (2004). *Consumer-directed health care: How well does it work?* Washington, DC: National Council on Disability. Retrieved from http://www.ncd.gov/newsroom/publications/2004/consumerdirected.htm

Patton, M. Q. (2002). *Qualitative evaluation and research methods* (3rd ed.). Thousand Oaks, CA: Sage.

Powers, L. E., Sowers, J., & Singer, G. H. S. (2006). A cross-disability analysis of person-directed, long-term services. *Journal of Disability Policy Studies*, *17*, 66–76.

President's New Freedom Commission on Mental Health. (2003). *Achieving the promise: Transforming mental health care in America*. Retrieved from http://www.mentalhealthcommission.gov/index.html

Rizzolo, M. C., Hemp, R., & Braddock, D. (2006). *Family support services in the United States* (Policy Research Brief 17). Minneapolis: University of Minnesota, Research and Training Center on Community Living.

Scala, M. A., Mayberry, P. S., & Kunkel, S. R. (1996). Consumer-directed home care: Client profiles and service challenges. *Journal of Case Management*, *5*, 91–98.

Shadish, W. R., Cook, T. D., & Campbell, D. T. (2002). *Experimental and quasi-experimental designs for generalized causal inference*. Boston: Houghton Mifflin.

Shevin, M., & Klein, N. (1984). The importance of choice-making skills for students with severe disabilities. *Journal of the Association for Persons with Severe Handicaps*, *9*, 159–166.

Simon-Rusinowitz, L., Mahoney, K. J., Loughlin, D. M., & Sadler, M. D. (2005). Paying family caregivers: An effective option in the Arkansas cash and counseling demonstration and evaluation. In R. K. Caputo (Ed.), *Challenges of aging on U.S. families: Policy and practice implications* (pp. 83–105). Binghamton, NY: Haworth.

Simon-Rusinowitz, L., Mahoney, K. J., Shoop, D. M., Desmond, S. M., Squillace, M. R., & Sowers, J. A. (2001). Consumer and surrogate preferences for a cash option versus transitional services: Florida adults with developmental disabilities. *Mental Retardation*, *39*, 87–103.

Velgouse, L., & Dize, V. (2000). A review of state initiatives in consumer-directed long-term care. *Generations*, *24*, 28–33.

Wehmeyer, M. L. (1998). Self-determination and individuals with significant disabilities: Examining meanings, and mis-interpretations. *Journal of the Association for Persons with Severe Handicaps*, *23*, 5–16.

Wood, W. M., Fowler, C. H., Uphold, N., & Test, D. W. (2005). A review of self-determination interventions with individuals with severe disabilities. *Research & Practice for Persons with Severe Disabilities*, *30*, 121–146.

Pediatric Disability and Caregiver Separation

JUDITH L. M. McCOYD, AYSE AKINCIGIL, and EUN KWANG PAEK

School of Social Work, Rutgers University, New Brunswick, New Jersey

The evidence that the birth of a child with a disability leads to divorce or separation is equivocal, with the majority of recent research suggesting that such a birth and childrearing may be stressful, but not necessarily toxic, to the caregiver relationship. Such research has been limited by small sample sizes and non-representative samples and has not been able to examine the caregivers' relationship stability over time. Using the National Survey of Supplemental Security Income (SSI) Children and Families (NSCF), data related to severity of the child's condition, caregiver burden, respite, and support group use were examined in relation to caregiver separation. Most variables showed no statistical significance. Our results did not support the hypothesis that the birth of a child with a disability leads to relationship dissolution. The instability of the child's condition and only extremely high levels of caregiver burden (the need for respite care and the need for the family to provide more than 48 hours of home health care) were positively associated with relationship separation. Use of a support group was associated with lower levels of relationship dissolution. The implications for service provision to families with a child living with disability are discussed. Additionally, because parental and practitioner culture often maintain the myth that the birth of a child with disability leads to dissolution of the caregiver relationship, implications of this are also addressed.

Judith L. M. McCoyd is grateful for a Research Council Grant from the Office of Research and Sponsored Programs, Rutgers University, the State University of New Jersey.

For years, practice wisdom held that parents who have a child born with a disability were at much higher risk for divorce or separation. Early research was often limited solely to an exploration of whether divorce followed the birth of a child with a disability. Despite this, families themselves have known that different families respond differently to the challenges involved in raising a child with a disabling condition. Some are able to find meaning in meeting the challenges involved in parenting a child with a disabling condition and find that it sensitizes them and their families to the human condition; others may fear those challenges and question their ability to meet their child's needs. Meanwhile, more recent studies, generally drawing data from small nonrepresentative samples, provide mixed results about the impact of the child's birth on the family. As current research begins examining moderating and mediating variables such as the impact of economic status and availability of resources, evidence about the impact on caregiver relationships has been equivocal. Nevertheless, a recent meta-analysis indicates that differences in marital distress are smaller than previous research would predict. Few of the previous studies have used large, nationally representative samples; and of those, even fewer have focused on identifying factors that appear to be protective or challenging to the caregiver relationship.

The current study, using a large, nationally representative sample of families who had experience with the Supplemental Security Income (SSI) program (National Survey of Supplemental Security Income Children and Families [NSCF]) at the time of first data collection in 1996 (with data collected again in 2000) attempts to rectify this. The current study explores factors that may be associated with separation/divorce among caregivers of children with disabilities and those that do not seem to be associated with increasing the likelihood of separation. Specific aims of the study are to

1. explore the impact of family caregiving and burden for children with disabilities on the stability of the caregiver's primary relationship (i.e., separation).
2. identify other risk or protective factors that are associated with separation.
3. examine association between the impact of family caregiving and burden and separation after controlling for the factors identified in Aim 2.

Working hypotheses included

Hypothesis 1: Families who face higher burden are more likely to experience caregiver separation than those who perceive less burden, that is, there is a positive linear relationship between caregiver burden and odds of separation.

Hypothesis 2: Families whose child is affected by greater levels of disability severity will have higher rates of separation, that is, there is a positive linear relationship between condition severity and odds of separation.

The SSI-NSCF data includes not only those who were approved to receive SSI for their child, but also those who applied and were above the income threshold or not deemed disabled "enough." This allows the generation of more generalizable findings, as well as contributing to the identification of factors that may promote the resiliency of families who are raising children with disabilities.

REVIEW OF THE LITERATURE

The U.S. Census Bureau (2000) reports that 6.55 million children who live in the United States have a diagnosable disability. Early research into the impact of having a child with a disabling condition indicated that divorce was a commonly seen outcome (Tew, Payne, & Laurence, 1974; Wolfensberger, 1967) despite evidence to the contrary in Great Britain (Hare, Laurence, Payne, & Rawnsley, 1966; Martin, 1975; Richards & McIntosh, 1973). Tew et al. (1974) asserted "that more often than not the family with a handicapped child is a handicapped family" (p. 97). They reported that divorce was significantly more likely among families with a child with a neural tube malformation ($n = 59$) compared to those whose child had no diagnosable abnormality ($n = 58$). Hare et al. (1966) also explored family experiences when a child was born with spina bifida but found little difference in marital dissolution. They asserted that marital stability within their group of 120 families was related to "depth of affection" and "maturity of personalities" (Hare et al., p. 758), not solely to the birth of the child with a disability. Richards and McIntosh (1973) hypothesized that poor social supports may contribute to marital difficulties more than the birth or disabling condition themselves. Despite these mixed results, the belief that the birth of a child with disabilities leads to marital stress and automatically leads to relationship dissolution is prevalent (Risdal & Singer, 2004).

It is true that all families are stressed when they add a new family member, even when this is due to an uncomplicated birth (Abidin, 1990), though others identify greater stresses on mothers when a child is born with a disability (Tobing & Glenwick, 2006). Some argue that the birth of a child with a disability is experienced in the same way as any birth; it is an event requiring major adjustments in roles, economic status, and relationships. Indeed, there are many who believe caregivers not only rise to the challenge of additional care but also benefit by virtue of heightened sensitivity, closer familial relationships, and opportunities for personal growth (Brown, 2008; Goodley & Tregaskis, 2006; Green, 2007; Morse, Wilson, & Penrod, 2000). Further, although findings have been mixed (Lundeby & Tossebro, 2008; Risdal & Singer, 2004; Swaminathan, Alexander, & Boulet, 2006; Urbano & Hodapp, 2007; Wymbs et al., 2008), the particular conditions causing disabilities seem to have little impact on marital stability after the second year of life (Starr, 1981; Swaminathan et al., 2006; Urbano & Hodapp, 2007).

Some, however, still report parental separation associated with children's poor health at birth, including (though not limited to) children born with disabilities (Reichman, Corman, & Noonan, 2004). Although poor health at birth differs from a lifetime lived with a disabling condition, these data have salience as the experience of raising a child from infancy to age 5 years may have many similarities between those born with ill health initially and children born with a disability. Our focus here is on these early years.

A recent meta-analysis conducted by Risdal and Singer (2004) found that marital distress was not dramatically increased due to raising a child with a disability. The use of meta-analysis allowed a synthesis of a broad range of studies from 1975 to 2003 that included some indicator of marital adjustment. Their finding of a detectable but small effect size indicates that the assumptions about negative impacts on parental relationships when a child is born with a disability are overstated.

Families raising children with disabilities are more likely to be living in poverty and/or under economic stress (Lukemeyer, Meyers, & Smeeding, 2000; Parish, Seltzer, Greenburg, & Floyd, 2004). Indeed, a recent report confirms previous findings that young children with disabilities are much more likely to live in poverty than children without disabilities (Parish & Cloud, 2006). Although giving birth tends to affect the income and time availability of women generally (Waldfogel, 1997), it is also apparent that the birth of a child with a disability has an even larger impact (MacInnes, 2008; Powers, 2001). It intuitively seems likely that parents stressed economically and socially by caring for children affected by disability may separate, yet beliefs that separation or divorce are highly correlated with this situation may not only be inaccurate but have far-reaching implications.

The vast majority of studies that examined relationship dissolution in connection to the birth of a child with a disability used divorce as the dependent variable rather than caregiver separation. The Reichman et al. study (2004) examined data from the Fragile Families and Child Wellbeing Study to investigate the father's presence in the home after 12 to 18 months. Although incorporating a larger sample than much of the previously cited research, their data were representative of a special segment of the population: nonmarital births in large urban cities in the United States. Although they are not constrained by official divorce as their dependent variable, the population is skewed. From Martin (1975) to Risdal and Singer (2004), many comment on the lack of large representative samples. There seems to be a reluctance to examine factors other than the mere existence of a child with a disability in the research exploring relationship stability. Yet parenting a child requiring more resources may be challenging, not so much because of the child's condition or direct impact on the relationship stability, as because of scarce resources for support.

In light of economic issues, resource availability seems to be an important factor to explore when examining how a family can manage the higher level of need that a child with a disabling condition has. The paucity of day care for children with disabilities and the difficulty finding other resources to assist with care means that many caretakers of children with the most severe disabilities report not being able to be part of the paid workforce due to responsibilities for child care (Leiter, Krauss, Anderson, & Wells, 2004). Lacking the income of the caregiver, even two-parent families struggle to meet the financial needs of their families, particularly the extra needs for equipment and supplies to help manage disabilities (Lukemeyer et al., 2000).

Decreases in income and limited care resources when parenting a child with a disabling condition create concrete pressures on caregivers. Psychosocial pressures exist as well. Caregiver burden seems to be affected by appraisal of the situation and degree of attachment to the child (Abidin, 1990), as well as approaches to parenting style (Woolfson & Grant, 2006). When appraisal of the situation is viewed as less stressful and attachment is higher, families may be better able to cope with additional expectations of care. In contrast, parents expecting to have a higher degree of control, as in the authoritative and authoritarian parenting styles (Baumrind, 1971; Woolfson & Grant, 2006), may lead to tensions between parental expectations and the child's abilities when affected by a disabling condition. This is in contrast with the typical parenting observations that authoritative parenting (a blend of firm guidance and warm nurturing) is the ideal type (Baumrind, 1971). Woolfson and Grant (2006) suggest that even authoritative parenting can put parents in conflict with children when they wish to control aspects of their child's behavior over which the child may have varying or little control.

Further, mothers and fathers may handle stress differently, which may or may not promote tensions between them due to discrepant perceptions of burden (Dyson, 1997). Interventions to provide support to such families and caregiver couples can be quite successful, when intervention includes work to ensure adequate respite for the caregivers and interpretation of caregiver stresses to promote cohesion rather than competition (Withers & Bennett, 2003). Although we are unable to examine parenting styles or appraisals, the association with perceived adequacy of available respite services is examined.

METHOD

Design, Data, and Study Population

The current study is a secondary analysis of public use data from NSCF, which collected data on children and young adults with special health care needs and their families who received or applied for SSI since 1978

(Mathematica Policy Research, 2004). The current study examines cross-sectional data collected between July 2001 and August 2002 for whom data were also collected in 1996. The study sample includes 8,726 respondents (generally parents) for children and young adults who had experience with the SSI program either as current or former beneficiaries or applicants who never received benefits. These data include SSI applicants as well as recipients and data capture multiple levels of disability, so the data is well suited to examine the hypotheses that there is a linear relationship between (1) caregiver burden and odds of separation and (2) condition severity and odds of separation.

The sampling frame consists of children and young adults in the SSI applicant and beneficiary files at two time points, December 1996 and December 2000. The NSCF used a complex probability sampling design, which was taken into account in the estimation procedures to derive appropriate standard deviation estimates. This public use data (PUD) included sampling weights which allowed researchers to obtain estimates of the Social Security Administration's (SSA's) national analytic populations and subpopulations. The weighted response rate for the NSCF was 74.4%, and the unweighted rate was 77.2%. Data collection was done with computer-assisted telephone and personal interviewing (CATI and CAPI). Details on sampling design and survey can be found at Mathematica Policy Research (2004). The objective of the current study is to describe couples' caregiving burden and its impact on relationship dissolution. Therefore the study population includes the married/cohabiting parents/guardians of children who were age 0 to 5 years in 1996. Relationship status in 1996 was based on self-report in the 2001 data collection. The question was worded: "In 1996, did you have a spouse or partner living with you?" The restrictions yielded a sample size of 1,123.

Measures

The binary outcome measure, dissolution of the relationship in 2001, was based on the survey item "Were you living with your current spouse or partner in 1996?" For purposes of the current study, separation of the parents/caregivers after a time of living together is the dependent variable. The data set does not consistently include marital status, but the separation variable is of more interest because it indicates that one caregiver has left the household and is therefore probably no longer readily available to assist with a dependent child's care. Explanatory variables include the severity of the child's condition, caregiver burden, and support group participation. Caregiver burden was measured by the services that a child needed: child's health care and medication needs ("does your child require more services/medication because of his/her current condition?" compared to typical children of the same age), use of respite care, and provision of home health care by family members (measured in hours). Variables related to the severity of the child's condition included the degree of limitation by disability compared to peers (reversely coded: 1 = *always*, 4 = *never*), the extent to which disability affected ability to do things (1 = *very little*, 3 = *a great deal*) and stability of health care needs (1 = *changed all the time*, 3 = *usually stable*).

Statistical Analyses

Univariate distributions describe the study population. To investigate the bivariate associations between independent variables (caregiver burden, condition severity, and support group participation) and dissolution of the relationship, we tabulated the rate of intact families in 2001 across independent variables. Bivariate associations were tested with the Pearson chi-square statistic. A probability of less than or equal to 0.05 resulted in rejecting the null hypothesis that the separation rates are unrelated to the explanatory variables. To better understand the relationship between independent variables and the likelihood of separation, a single multivariate logistic regression model was estimated predicting the probability of "staying intact." The binary dependent variable was coded as 1 for families that stayed intact and 0 for families that separated. All covariates (caregiver burden, condition severity, and support group participation) were included on the right-hand side to minimize the possibility of omitted variable bias. Estimated regression coefficients were converted into odds ratios (ORs), reporting odds of staying intact in the referred group to the odds of it occurring in the reference group. We also reported the 95% confidence intervals for these ORs. For each coefficient estimate, we reported the Wald chi-square statistic and its probability value, testing the statistical significance of each predictor against the null that OR is equal to one, all else equal, that is, holding the other predictors constant. Unless stated as "sample size," all analyses are weighted, and standard errors were calculated with survey procedures that take the sampling design into account (i.e., svy: tabulate, and svy: logistic procedures in STATA/SE version 9.2 were used).

RESULTS

Medication and service utilization was common in the population (see Table 1); 63% required more services ($n = 825$) and 53% required more medications ($n = 562$), according to parental perceptions about their child's needs in contrast to what has been received. There is large variation in caregiver burden: Almost two thirds of the population did not require home health care (62%, $n = 629$), 15% required 1 to 4 hours of care per week, 4% required 5 to 12 hours of home care per week, 13% required 13 to 47 hours per week, and a small proportion (6%) required extremely intense care

TABLE 1 Description of Child's Condition, Caregiver Burden, Participation in the Support Groups and Relationship Status

	Sample size	Population ratio (%)[b]
All[a]	1,123	100
Caregiver burden		
Require more services		
No	298	36.0
Yes	825	63.0
Require more medications		
No	481	47.1
Yes	642	52.9
Provision of home health care[c]		
None	629	62.4
1–4 Hours Per Week	126	15.1
5–12 Hours Per Week	96	3.7
13–47 Hours Per Week	120	12.9
>48 Hours Per Week	100	5.9
Require respite care[d]		
No	822	83.5
Yes	202	16.5
Severity of child's condition		
Limitation compared to peers[e]		
Never/sometimes	576	61.1
Usually/always	528	38.9
Disability affects ability to do things[f]		
A great deal	348	25.5
Some	481	42.5
Very little	272	32.0
Stability of health care needs[g]		
Change all the time	227	18.2
Change only once in a while	399	34.1
Usually stable	445	47.8
Support group participation		
No	746	70.2
Yes	377	29.8
Relationship status in 2001		
Separated (0)	417	36.5
Intact (1)	706	63.5

Note: [a]Study population includes the married/cohabiting parents/guardians of SSI children that were aged 0–5 in 1996.

[b]Weighted, reflect national estimates.

[c]By the parent(s)/guardian(s); missing for 52 cases.

[d]Missing for 99 cases.

[e]Missing for 19 cases.

[f]Missing for 22 cases.

[g]Missing for 52 cases.

(>48 hours of home health care per week). In addition, another 17% ($n = 202$) required respite care.

Almost 4 out of 10 children were reported to have high levels of limitation compared to peers (39%, $n = 528$). Among one fourth, the child's ability to do things was affected "a great deal," whereas among 32%, the child's ability to do things was minimally affected. Almost one half of the children's health care needs were generally stable; meanwhile, for 18% the health care needs "changed all the time." Almost 30% of the couples participated in support groups ($n = 377$).

The majority of the families were intact in 2001 (63.5%, $n = 706$, Table 2). The first two columns of Table 2 present the results of the bivariate analyses with Pearson's chi-square; the remaining columns present the OR and Wald chi-square results and their significance as derived from the logistic regression model, F (13, 558) = 9.70, probability $> F = 0.0001$. Separation rates did not vary significantly by medication and service needs of the child. With the exception of the children that require extreme intensity of home health care (>48 hours per week), separation rates actually declined as the child's need for home health care needs increased ($p = 0.043$). For example, of the families with children who do not require home health care, 60% remained intact, compared to 73% to 74% among the families that provide home health care between 5 to 47 hours per week (yielding ORs of 73% intact for 5–12 hours; and 74% for 12–47 hours, respectively). Even among the parents who provide very intense levels of care (48+ hours/week), intact rates were higher, compared with the families that do not provide care (63% vs. 60%). Among the parents of the children who require respite care, rates of staying intact were 59% versus 65% among the parents of children that do not require such care. Although the bivariate difference was not statistically significant, multivariate analyses confirmed the direction and significance of the findings. Once all other covariates were controlled for, parents of children who require respite care (according to the caregivers' perception) had statistically significantly lower odds of staying intact. This difference may mirror the finding of higher levels of dissolution when caregivers are stressed to an extreme level, as families providing 48 hours/week of care would seem to indicate.

Neither rates nor odds of staying intact were significantly associated with the child's limitations or the effect of disability on the child's ability to do things. Meanwhile, degree of variation in the child's health care needs had a large impact on rates and odds of separation. Compared to the children with usually stable health care needs, parents that face the largest variation (health care needs "change all the time") were half as likely to remain intact (OR = 0.49), after controlling for the characteristics of the child's condition and caregiving burden. We observed a smaller but still significant effect among families of children whose health care needs change once in a while as well, compared to usually stable (OR = 0.74). Finally, support group participation was associated with increased likelihood of staying intact in 5 years, after controlling for the child's condition and caregiver burden (OR = 1.48).

TABLE 2 Proportion of Families that Stayed Intact and Logistic Regression Model Results

	Chi-square results		Logistic regression model results	
	% intact[b]	*p* value	Odds ratio[c] (95% confidence interval)	Wald chi-square statistic and *p* value
All[a]	63.5			
Caregiver Burden				
Require more services		0.793		
No (Reference)	64.3		1.00	–
Yes	63.1		1.02 (0.84, 1.26)	0.25 (0.806)
Require more medications		0.701		
No (Reference)	64.3		1.00	–
Yes	62.8		0.96 (0.80, 1.15)	−0.43 (0.671)
Provision of home health care		0.043		
None (Reference)	60.3		1.00	–
1–4 Hours Per Week	67.3		1.40 (1.04, 1.88)[d]	2.23 (0.026)
5–12 Hours Per Week	73.2		1.99 (1.46, 2.73)[d]	4.29 (0.001)
13–47 Hours Per Week	74.3		1.34 (0.98, 1.83)[d]	1.83 (0.067)
>48 Hours Per Week	63.1		1.42 (1.09, 1.83)[d]	2.65 (0.008)
Require Respite Care		0.174		
No (Reference)	64.5		1.00	–
Yes	58.8		0.75 (0.62, 0.90)[d]	−3.08 (0.002)
Severity of child's condition				
Limitation compared to peers		0.309		
Never/sometimes (Reference)	65.0		1.00	–
Usually/always	61.0		1.07 (0.87, 1.32)	0.68 (0.497)
Disability affects ability to do things		0.600		
A great deal	66.0		1.10 (0.81, 1.50)	0.64 (0.521)
Some	61.3		1.03 (0.80, 1.32)	0.26 (0.798)
Very little (Reference)	63.8		1.00	–
Stability of health care needs		0.517		
Change all the time	58.3		0.49 (0.40, 0.60)[d]	−6.76 (0.001)
Change only once in a while	63.0		0.74 (0.63, 0.87)[d]	−3.66 (0.001)
Usually stable (Reference)	65.5		1.00	–
Support group participation				
No (Reference)	61.6	0.139	1.00	–
Yes	68.1		1.48 (1.23, 1.79)[d]	4.14 (0.001)

Note: [a]Study population includes the married/cohabiting parents/guardians of SSI children that were age 0 to 5 years in 1996.

[b]Population ratio (rates are weighted and standard errors were calculated with survey procedures that take the sampling design into account).

[c]Based on logistic regression where the dependent variable is the binary outcome indicating separation in 2001.

[d]Odds ratio is significantly different than one at 95% level of confidence.

Model statistics: $F(13, 558) = 9.70$. Prob. $> F = 0.0001$.

DISCUSSION

Findings from the NSCF indicate few statistically significant associations between variables related to caregiver burden and the severity of the child's condition and the dependent variable of relationship dissolution/separation. Neither of the hypotheses was supported by the data. This large nationally representative sample allows us to reexamine negative assumptions about the impact of children with disabilities on their families. Our analysis of the evidence supports the growing body of knowledge that relationship stability is not automatically compromised upon the birth of a child with a disability, yet there are important nuances to this finding. Although there is not a linear relationship between the severity of the child's condition or caregiver burden and relationship dissolution, other factors related to stability of the child's condition, need for caregivers to provide extensive home health care, and the need for respite show significance.

In this sample, (i.e., families with children with special health care needs who received or applied for SSI), 64% of the families were intact after 5 years of the child's birth. Although separation is the dependent variable, the closest comparable national statistic is divorce rates. Because divorce rates vary considerably from state to state (Munson & Sutton, 2004) and among demographic groups (Kreider & Fields, 2001; Popenoe, 2007), it is difficult to compare rates of separation or divorce among families with a child with a disability and comparable families raising typical children. In their analyses of nonmarital births in large urban cities in the United States, Reichman et al. (2004) reported that 63% of the parents live together within 12 to 18 months after birth. In that sample, 5% of the sample consisted of children with poor health. The U.S. Census Bureau (2000) report indicates that information regarding marriage and divorce is difficult to estimate since the suspension of collection of marriage and divorce statistics in 1996 by the National Center for Health Statistics. Nevertheless, they project that nearly one half of first marriages for individuals younger than age 45 may end in divorce (Kreider & Fields, 2001). Given the preponderance of this evidence, it seems our sample is well within customary rates of separation for families with younger children and other families under some degree of stress (therefore not necessarily due to the birth of a child with a disability).

When considering the child's level of disability, we used proxies. When the child required more services or more medication, they were assumed to have higher levels of disability, yet neither of these predicted a significant impact on relationship stability. Likewise, the caregiver reported assessment that the child was usually more limited than his or her peers or that the disability affects the child's ability to do things even "a great deal of the time" were also not found to be associated in a significant way with relationship dissolution.

The hours of home health care provided by the family provides an interesting trend for further examination. It appears that the need for family provision of home health care decreases the likelihood of separation until it hits the extreme of 48 hours per week or more. Even at that point, the percentage of intact families is higher than for families who do not need to provide such care (63% in contrast to 60%, a nonsignificant difference). There appears to be some support for a hypothesis that lesser degrees of stress (but some) are actually perceived in ways that may promote remaining intact, at least up to a threshold beyond which the stress is too great for the relationship to tolerate.

Yet when caregivers perceive need for respite care (likely a proxy for high level of severity and/or burden), the likelihood of separation increases significantly. This may also be consistent with the finding of the case study by Withers and Bennett (2003) that availability of respite care provides crucial time for the parents/caregivers to attend to their own relationship and to have time where they are not "on-call" constantly. This is a major concern in a country where cuts in social services due to economic downturns are widespread. Respite care is often one of the first areas to be cut because it is assumed that, if the child is living with a two-parent family, the family will be able to continue to provide care. The current study suggests that a felt need for respite care may be one of the crucial factors in taking a family able to maintain its stability into the danger zone where the stress outweighs the family's ability to cope. Yet prior research has shown that informal caregivers are often hesitant to express a need for respite services (Van Exel, de Graaf, & Brouwer, 2008), though this finding is from the Netherlands where norms about use of social care services may differ somewhat. Nevertheless, in the United States, practitioners report parents often feel guilt for availing themselves of respite rather than acknowledging it as "an essential, not a luxury" (Orloff, 2007, p. 69).

Further, uncertainty seems to be a critical stressor as indicated by the increasing percentage of couples who separate in the face of the child's health condition "chang[ing] all the time" (0.49 (0.40,0.60*); 58% intact vs. 65.5% intact for "usually stable"). Taken together, these findings also point toward a theory that a certain degree of stress (i.e., the child's diagnosis with a disability and some level of need that the caregivers feel capable of meeting) works in protective ways for the relationship (possibly by bringing the adults closer together due to a shared goal but also possibly due to a sense that one has fewer options for separating). It seems that after a certain threshold of severity and caregiver burden, the likelihood of dissolution increases, theoretically due to higher levels of individual and couple stressors.

According to a large study on marital disruption, a primary factor in marital dissolution is the woman's sense of being "underbenefitted," meaning that she feels as if she gets few benefits from maintaining the relationship (Demaris, 2007). This situation may be less likely if a mother (or primary caregiver) is caring for a disabled child and the other caregiver is helping economically with the child's care. When she is supported in these endeavors, there may be more willingness to maintain and even thrive within the relationship. Further, evidence from families with children with attention-deficit hyperactivity disorder suggests that, when the second parent is unavailable for assistance due to his or her own mental health or other issues (yet is physically present in the household), divorce is more likely (Wymbs et al., 2008). Bristol, Gallagher, and Schopler (1988) examined the impact on families of a son with a developmental disability in contrast to those with no disability (all families were White). They found that fathers typically had fewer responsibilities and caretaking with their sons who had disabilities, not just in contrast with fathers with typically developing sons, but also in contrast with their care of other children in the home. Crucially, there was a level of "harmonic" support between parenting couples when the fathers' proffered support met the needs and expectations of the mother. Participation of both partners in support of the child's needs, as well as each other, seems to be crucial in protecting the caregiver relationship.

It is notable that, although only a one-fourth to one-third of families participated in a support group, the participation was associated with lower separation rates (68.1% intact with an OR = 1.48, CI 1.23, 1.79*). Obviously, we cannot make any causal inferences; it is possible, though, that the support group may be helping the couples, or it is possible that the couples that choose to receive support services are systematically different from the others, a difference that also affects their likelihood of separation. Still, it needs to be noted that this finding is consistent with the theory that the mere existence of a child with a disability in the family is not the factor that influences the relationship stability as much as the degree of stress experienced by the caregivers. When caregivers receive the support of a support group, and/or discover that they have issues much like other families in similar circumstances, they may be able to develop a perspective where the partner is viewed as part of the solution rather than part of the problem. Even where a child is severely affected (disability affects ability to do things), the family does not have higher odds of separation after controlling for other variables. The lack of stability of the child's health is likely influential because there is little ability to develop a care routine and the primary caregiver may feel "underbenefitted" on a regular basis when the child's condition requires more care, but the caregiving routine does not include enough support. Support groups may also assist the family in normalizing the experience of incorporating a family member with greater than average needs for care (Morse et al., 2000).

It is notable that the research here is consistent with the meta-analysis by Risdal and Singer (2004) who challenged four assumptions: first, that the birth of a child with a disability causes only distress (with no identification of family strengths); second, that family distress was caused by the fact of the child's condition rather than other mediating or moderating variables; third, that there was little variability among families; and fourth, that the family stress was immutable. Our findings also challenge the idea that families experience only distress because there was no significant difference in relationship dissolution overall. Further, there are strong indications that variables such as respite provision, hours of home care required of the caregivers, and support group use may affect the caregiver relationship. This also shows that there is a level of variability among families and implies that appropriate supports may act in a protective manner to enable families to maintain stability. Further research is necessary to tease out the psychosocial attachment and appraisal factors' impact, as well as to explore how the use of home care, respite care, and support groups may mediate or moderate relationship stressors and/or the stability of the relationship.

There are other, more distant implications of these findings. As a clinician working with families around perinatal and pediatric deaths, one author (JM) had many mentors who repeated the belief that death of a child would lead to divorce as a "given" of practice with this population. Yet in 1998, Schwab asserted that "It is time for professionals to dispel that myth" (p. 445). She cited others who had found that the rates of divorce were not significantly greater than the rise in divorces in the population more generally. Certainly, findings that divorce rates were not significantly increased should not be interpreted to mean that bereaved parents are not stressed individually and as a couple, nor that they may not benefit greatly from the support of social workers and others. Yet perpetuation of the myth may lead to unwarranted additional concern about the potential health of the relationship at a time when vulnerability and pain are already present after a child's death.

Likewise, when women receive the results of prenatal diagnostic tests that they are at higher risk for fetal anomalies, the findings from the current study may have great salience. The same mentors for perinatal practice mentioned above repeated the assertion that the birth of a child with a disability would also lead to divorce. Indeed, in a recent study, many women cited fears of separation and divorce as part of the reason for terminating pregnancies affected by fetal anomaly (McCoyd, 2003, 2008). Advances in prenatal testing have occurred quickly, enabling women and couples to make choices about whether to continue a pregnancy where the fetus is diagnosed with a disability/anomaly and thereby forcing them to grapple with decision making that has ethical, economic, and emotional consequences (McCoyd, 2003, 2007, 2009). Decisions about whether to continue a pregnancy affected by a fetal anomaly most frequently occur under conditions of uncertainty about individual levels of risk for fetal anomaly (as risk is given as a statistical function) and uncertainty about level of functional impairment of the fetus if brought to birth (Lawson, 2001; Schectman, Gray, Baty, & Rothman, 2002).

These decisions are also predicated on an understanding about the impact of raising a child with a disability (McCoyd, 2008), an understanding often informed by opinion as well as fact. When parents rely on the belief that the birth of a child with a disability will lead to divorce or separation, they are relying upon a myth, incomplete and inaccurate information.

This is critical because people may rely on this information and may terminate a pregnancy based primarily on an inaccurate belief rather than upon a full assessment of the challenges (and possible benefits) that giving birth to a child with a disability may entail.

Additionally, the belief that relationship instability or dissolution comes as a result of a child being born with a disability relieves policy makers of the responsibility to identify social supports that would enable families to be more stable. When relationship instability can be attributed to the birth itself, few look further to identify the services that are needed. When home care, respite, and support groups are provided at adequate levels, particularly when the health care needs of the child change frequently, they may be protective of the relationship. Policy makers who wish to assist families in maintaining their ability to support children with disabling conditions would be wise to heed the need for these services before the child becomes the primary responsibility of a single parent who may be even more stressed by care giving needs.

Limitations to the current study include the fact that the data do not allow for more in-depth exploration of the caregiver's perceptions of the quality of the relationship before and after a dissolution, nor are there data relating to their attributions about the reason/s for the separation. There is also no data on attachment of the caregiver to the child, or appraisal of the levels of stress on the individual caregiver or the caregivers' relationship, meaning that these variables, found to be significant in other small studies, were not able to be examined. The data also lack extensive information about economic stressors. As a nationwide, longitudinal study utilizing probability sampling, generalization is limited to those who have made the connection with the SSA to apply for supplemental income and do not reflect those families where use of governmental services is limited, either due to not applying for SSI due to too much family income, or due to immigration status. Further, the data is all self-report and is therefore affected by recall bias, desirability bias, and other common biases of self-report studies. Further, the data support correlational findings, but randomized trials providing different support services will help to identify which services help to improve outcomes for the child directly, as well as how those supports may affect family stability.

CONCLUSIONS

Families raising children with disabilities are challenged by economic and caregiving burdens, yet there is little support for the belief that the birth of a disabled child raises the risk of parental/caregiver separation. Analysis of separation among caregivers for children with disabilities who have applied for (and often received) SSI indicates that the presence of a disability, even a relatively severe one, has less detrimental impact on the relationship than instability of the child's condition and/or the felt need for further levels of care (i.e., high levels of needed home care, need for respite). Further, support group participation may be protective, leading to significantly less likelihood of separation. The need to ensure appropriate supports for home health care and emotional support for family members remains strong for families with disabled children, yet if these needs are met adequately, there is evidence that the relationship will survive. Policy makers must not believe the myth that the birth of a child with a disability is what leads to relationship dissolution; they, like parents and practitioners, must understand that families benefit when supports are available to assist with stressors.

REFERENCES

Abidin, R. R. (1990). Introduction to the special issue: The stresses of parenting. *Journal of Clinical Child Psychology*, *19*(4), 298–301.

Baumrind, D. (1971). Current patterns of parental authority. *Developmental Psychology Monograph*, *4*, 1–103.

Bristol, M. M., Gallagher, J. J., & Schopler, E. (1988). Mothers and fathers of young developmentally disabled and nondisabled boys: Adaptation and spousal support. *Developmental Psychology*, *24*(3), 441–451.

Brown, J. D. (2008). Rewards of fostering children with disability. *Journal of Family Social Work*, *11*(1), 36–49.

Demaris, A. (2007). The role of relationship inequity in marital disruption. *Journal of Social and Personal Relationships*, *24*(2), 177–195.

Dyson, L. L. (1997). Fathers and mothers of school-age children with developmental disabilities: Parental stress, family functioning, and social support. *American Journal on Mental Retardation*, *102*(3), 267–279.

Goodley, D., & Tragaskis, C. (2006). Storying disability and impairment: Retrospective accounts of disabled family life. *Qualitative Health Research*, *16*(5), 630–646.

Green, S. E. (2007). "We're tired, not sad": Benefits and burdens of mothering a child with a disability. *Social Science and Medicine*, *64*, 150–163.

Hare, E. H., Laurence, K. M., Payne, H., & Rawnsley, K. (1966). Spina bifida cystica and family stress. *British Medical Journal*, *2*, 757–760. doi:10.1136/bmj.2.5516.757

Kreider, R. M., & Fields, J. M. (2001). Number, timing and duration of marriages and divorces: Fall 1996. *Current Population Reports*, 70–80. Retrieved August 31, 2009, from http://www.census.gov/prod/2002pubs/p70-80.pdf

Lawson, K. L. (2001). Contemplating selective reproduction: the subjective appraisal of parenting a child with a disability. *Journal of Reproductive and Infant Psychology*, *19*(1), 73–82.

Leiter, V., Krauss, M. W., Anderson, B., & Wells, N. (2004). The consequences of caring: Effects of mothering a child with special needs. *Journal of Family Issues*, *25*, 379–403.

Lukemeyer, A., Meyers, M. K., & Smeeding, T. (2000). Expensive children in poor families: Out-of-pocket expenditures for the care of disabled and chronically ill children in welfare families. *Journal of Marriage and the Family*, *62*, 399–415.

Lundeby, H., & Tossebro, J. (2008). Family structure in Norwegian families of children with disabilities. *Journal of Applied Research in Intellectual Disabilities*, *21*(3), 246–256.

Martin, P. (1975). Marital breakdown in families of patients with spina bifida cystica. *Developmental Medicine and Child Neurology*, *17*(6), 757–764.

Mathematica Policy Research, Inc. (2004). *National Survey of SSI Children and Families User's Manual for Restricted and Public Use Files* (Gillcrist, J. & Edson, D.). Retrieved June 13, 2006, from http://www.ssa.gov/disabilityresearch/nscf.htm

MacInnes, M. D. (2008). One's enough for now: Children, disability, and the subsequent childbearing of mothers. *Journal of Marriage and the Family*, *70*(3), 758–771.

McCoyd, J. L. M. (2003). *Pregnancy interrupted: Non-normative loss of a desired pregnancy after termination for fetal anomaly* [dissertation]. Bryn Mawr, PA: Bryn Mawr College. Available from Proquest (UMI No. 3088602).

McCoyd, J. L. M. (2007). Pregnancy interrupted: Loss of a desired pregnancy after diagnosis of fetal anomaly. *Journal of Psychosomatic Obstetrics and Gynecology*, *28*(1), 37–48.

McCoyd, J. L. M. (2008). I'm not a saint: Burden assessment as an unrecognized factor in prenatal decision making. *Qualitative Health Research*, *18*(11), 1489–1500.

McCoyd, J. L. M. (2009). Discrepant feeling rules and unscripted emotion work: Women terminating desired pregnancies due to fetal anomaly. *American Journal of Orthopsychiatry*, *79*(4), 441–451.

Morse, J. M., Wilson, S., & Penrod, J. (2000). Mothers and their disabled children: Refining the concept of normalization. *Health Care for Women International*, *21*, 659–676.

Munson, M. L., & Sutton, P. D. (2004). Births, marriages, divorces, and deaths: National provisional data for 2003. *National Vital Statistics Report*, *52*(22). Retrieved August 15, 2009, from http://www.cdc.gov/nchs/data/nvsr/nvsr52.htm

Orloff, S. S. (2007). Respite care: An essential, not a luxury! *Exceptional Parent*, *37*, 69.

Parish, S. L., & Cloud, J. M. (2006). Financial well-being of young children with disabilities and their families. *Social Work*, *51*(3), 223–232.

Parish, S. L., Seltzer, M. M., Greenberg, J. S., & Floyd, F. J. (2004). Economic implications of caregiving at midlife: Comparing parents of children with developmental disabilities to other parents. *Mental Retardation*, *4*(6), 413–426.

Popenoe, D. (2007). *The state of our unions 2007: The social health of marriage in America*. Piscataway, NJ: The National Marriage Project.

Powers, E. T. (2001). New estimates of the impact of child disability on maternal employment. *American Economic Review*, *91*, 135–139.

Reichman, N. E., Corman, H., & Noonan, K. (2004). Effects of child health on parents' relationship status. *Demography*, *41*(3), 569–584.

Richards, I. D. G., & McIntosh, H. T. (1973). Spinal bifida survivors and their parents: a study of problems and services. *Developmental Medicine and Child Neurology*, *15*(3), 292–304.

Risdal, D., & Singer, G. H. S. (2004). Marital adjustment in parents of children with disabilities: A historical review and meta-analysis. *Research and Practice for Persons with Severe Disabilities*, *29*(2), 95–103.

Schectman, K. B., Gray, D. L., Baty, J. D., & Rothman, S. M. (2002). Decision-making for termination of pregnancies with fetal anomalies: Analysis of 53,000 pregnancies. *Obstetrics and Gynecology*, *99*(2), 216–222.

Schwab, R. (1998). A child's death and divorce: Dispelling the myth. *Death Studies*, *22*, 445–468.

Starr, P. (1981). Marital status and raising a handicapped child: Does one affect the other? *Social Work*, *6*(4), 504–506.

Swaminathan, S., Alexander, G. R., & Boulet, S. (2006). Delivering a very low birth weight infant and the subsequent risk of divorce or separation. *Maternal and Child Health Journal*, *10*(6), 473–479.

Tew, B. J., Payne, H., & Laurence, K. M. (1974). Must a family with a handicapped child be a handicapped family? *Developmental Medicine and Child Neurology*, *16*(32), 95–98.

Tobing, L. E., & Glenwick, D. S. (2006). Predictors and moderators of psychological distress in mothers of children with pervasive developmental disorders. *Journal of Family Social Work*, *10*(4), 1–20.

Urbano, R. C., & Hodapp, R. M. (2007). Divorce in families of children with Down syndrome: A population-based study. *American Journal on Mental Retardation*, *112*(4), 261–274.

U.S. Census Bureau. (2000). *Disability statistics*. Retrieved August 20, 2009, from http://www.census.gov/hhes/www/disability/data_title.html#2000

Van Exel, J., de Graaf, G., & Brouwer, W. (2008). Give me a break! Informal caregiver attitudes towards respite care. *Health Policy*, *88*, 73–87.

Waldfogel, J. (1997). The effect of children on women's wages. *American Sociological Review*, *62*, 209–217.

Withers, P., & Bennett, L. (2003). Myths and marital discord in a family with a child with profound physical and intellectual disabilities. *British Journal of Learning Disabilities*, *31*, 91–95.

Wolfensberger, W. (1967). Counseling the parents of the retarded. In B. A. Baumeister (Ed.), *Mental retardation: Appraisal, education and rehabilitation* (pp. 329–400). Chicago: Aldine.

Woolfson, L., & Grant, E. (2006). Authoritative parenting and parental stress in parents of pre-school and older children with developmental disabilities. *Child: Care, Health & Development*, *32*(2), 177–184.

Wymbs, B. T., Pelham, W.E., Molina, B. S. G., Gnagy, E. M., Wilson, T. K., & Greenhouse, J. B. (2008). Rate and predictors of divorce among parents of youths with ADHD. *Journal of Consulting and Clinical Psychology*, *76*(5), 735–744.

Latina Mothers Caring for a Son or Daughter With Autism or Schizophrenia: Similarities, Differences, and the Relationship Between Co-Residency and Maternal Well-Being

SANDY MAGAÑA and SUBHARATI GHOSH

School of Social Work, University of Wisconsin–Madison, Madison, Wisconsin

In this cross-sectional study, the authors examined similarities and differences in depressive symptoms and psychological well-being between Latina maternal caregivers of persons with autism (n = 29) and schizophrenia (n = 33). They also explored predictors of maternal outcomes and the relationship of co-residence to them. Regression analysis found that mothers of adults with schizophrenia had lower levels of psychological well-being than mothers of youth or adults with autism. For the overall sample of mothers, co-residing with their son or daughter was significantly related to lower levels of depressive symptoms. Qualitative analysis of the nine mothers who lived apart from their son or daughter revealed that extreme behavior problems of the son or daughter and poor maternal health contributed to living apart. Despite overcoming these challenges, mothers expressed a profound sense of sadness about their sons' or daughters' living arrangements.

It is important to examine the experiences of Latino caregivers across disability contexts to determine whether and how these experiences may differ depending on the diagnosis of the child. Latinos have become the largest

Research for this article was supported by R01-MH55928 (Jan Seven Greenberg, PhD, PI) from the National Institute of Mental Health (NIMH), and R01-AG08768 (Marsha Mailick Seltzer, PhD, PI) from the National Institute on Aging (NIA). The authors wish to give a special acknowledgment to the families who participated in their study.

minority group in the United States (Cohn, 2003) and are very likely to be intimately involved with caring for family members with disabilities across the life span. Although there is a moderate amount of research on Latino caregivers of older adults with dementia and other disabilities (Magaña, 2006), this article focuses on Latina mothers who care for their own youth or adult children with one of two neurological disorders—autism and schizophrenia. This is a topic that has not received much attention in the literature. We explore whether maternal depressive symptoms and psychological well-being differ between the two groups of mothers, what the overall predictors are, and the relationship between coresidency and maternal well-being.

CAREGIVING IN AUTISM AND MENTAL ILLNESS

There are many aspects that are different about caring for a son or daughter with autism and caring for a son or daughter with schizophrenia that are important to consider. Age of diagnosis is one distinct difference; autism is typically diagnosed between the ages of 2 and 5 years, and schizophrenia is diagnosed in adolescence and young adulthood. Thus the timing of diagnosis occurs in different stages of the parents' life course, early adulthood for parents of children with autism and midlife for parents of children with schizophrenia (Greenberg, Seltzer, Krauss, Chou, & Hong, 2004). Not only is the life stage of the parents different between the two, but also the life stage of the child is different, which may affect the parent's perspective and acceptance of the child. A diagnosis such as autism or schizophrenia may be difficult to accept at first for any parent. Receiving the diagnosis when the child is young, as is the case with autism, may influence maternal perception and acceptance of that child differently than if the child had grown up normally and then changed in behavior and character, as is frequently the case with schizophrenia. For autism and schizophrenia, behavior problems of the son or daughter may challenge parental caregivers. Behavior problems and symptoms for children with autism can be severe but tend to decrease into adulthood (Shattuck et al., 2007). In contrast, behavior problems in schizophrenia can be less predictable and often occur in cycles (American Psychiatric Association [APA], 2000).

With respect to behavior problems, it is important to differentiate behaviors from symptoms and understand how they relate to each diagnostic group. For autism, core symptoms involve impaired development in reciprocal social interaction and communication, and restricted and repetitive behaviors (APA, 2000). Behavior problems may develop from the interaction of these core symptoms with family and societal expectations. For example, the child may become frustrated by the inability to communicate well or may be averse to social and other stimulation, thus reacting in a negative way. People with schizophrenia may manifest positive or negative symptoms (APA, 2000). Positive symptoms are those that are seen as overtly psychotic such as experiencing hallucinations or delusions. As a result of these symptoms, the person may exhibit what are seen as strange behaviors that can be offensive to others or embarrassing to caregivers. Negative symptoms include inability to initiate or sustain goal-directed activities, poverty of speech, and flat affect (APA, 2000). These symptoms can be seen as problematic for caregivers who would like their son or daughter to be more active in becoming independent in their own life goals. The behavior problems that result from symptoms interacting with the social environment may be very similar across both groups. For example both groups may exhibit behaviors such as hurting oneself or others, embarrassing caregivers in public, or being uncooperative or offensive in public.

Some of the similarities between the two groups allow for comparison because variables that are difficult to measure are more likely to remain constant between the two groups. For example, both of these groups experience hardships in the diagnostic process because diagnosis is based on a behavioral assessment as opposed to a genetic or biological test and may experience stress as a result of their "diagnostic odyssey" (Seltzer, Abbeduto, Krauss, Greenberg, & Swe, 2004). In addition, there is some evidence among both groups of caregivers that there is an elevated genetic risk for psychiatric problems such as depression; therefore, comparisons between these two groups may control for these potential genetic predispositions (Seltzer, Abbeduto et al., 2004).

Other similarities between caregivers of persons with autism and schizophrenia include the quality of relationships between parent and child and that this relationship is significant in predicting parental well-being (Greenberg et al., 2004). Because of social impairments in both groups, the quality of relationship between the sons or daughter sand their parental caregivers may be affected. A study that compared mothers of adults with autism to mothers of adults with schizophrenia found no differences in either quality of relationship or level of caregiver optimism (Greenberg et al., 2004). These researchers also found that better quality relationships were related to higher levels of optimism and better well-being outcomes for both groups. Additionally, they found that there were no differences in depressive symptoms or psychological well-being between the two groups of caregivers (Greenberg et al., 2004). Research has been mixed on whether there are differences in well-being outcomes among caregivers of adults with intellectual disabilities (ID) and caregivers of adults with mental illness (Greenberg, Seltzer, & Greenley, 1993; Seltzer, Greenberg, Floyd, & Hong, 2004); however, so far, researchers who have examined differences between caregivers of adults with autism and schizophrenia have found more similarities than differences in caregiver outcomes. Although these studies demonstrate emerging data on how these two groups may be similar, there has been no research examining these two groups of caregivers together among Latino families; and little research of Latino caregivers of persons with mental illness or autism at all.

RESEARCH ON LATINA MOTHERS OF CHILDREN/ADULTS WITH INTELLECTUAL DISABILITIES (ID) AND MENTAL ILLNESS

Latina mothers of children with disabilities, similar to mothers in other minority groups, may be faced with challenges associated with low socioeconomic status (SES) such as poor housing, poor health, and limited access to health insurance and resources. Recent research has found that Latina and African American mothers who care for adult children with schizophrenia and children or adults with ID are more likely to suffer from poorer health and higher rates of psychological distress than their noncaregiving peers (Blacher, Lopez, Shapiro, & Fusco, 1997; Magaña, Greenberg, & Seltzer, 2004; Magaña & Smith, 2006a). Differences in health and psychological distress between non-Latino caregivers of adult children with ID and parents whose children do not have these same disabilities have not been found (Seltzer, Greenberg, Floyd, Pettee, & Hong, 2001); however, these differences have been found between non-Latina mothers of adults with mental illness and mothers whose children do not have mental illness (Seltzer et al., 2004). These findings suggest a cumulative effect of caregiving on health that may have a greater impact on some mothers as they age.

Although there are different countries of origin for Latinos, with distinct political histories, practices, and customs, there is some evidence that cultural values and practices related to the family may provide a common experience for many Latino caregivers (Aranda & Knight, 1997). For example, within-group studies have found that Latino caregivers of persons with mental illness or ID tend to rely on family members for advice and support (Blacher et al., 1997; Guarnaccia & Parra, 1996; Magaña, 1999). Informal social support networks of caregivers of adults with an ID tend to consist primarily of family members, and size of and satisfaction with social support networks have been found to be significantly related to caregiver well-being (Magaña, 1999).

Latino youth and adults with an ID or mental illness are more likely to live with their parents than non-Latino White persons with these disabilities (Heller, Markwardt, Rowitz, & Farber, 1994; Magaña & Smith, 2006b; Milstein, Guarnaccia, & Midlarsky, 1995). Studies find that around 75% of Latino caregivers coreside with their son or daughter with autism or mental illness compared to 33% to 45% among non-Latino White families (Greenberg et al., 2004; Heller et al., 1994; Magaña, Garcia, Hernández, & Cortez, 2007; Milstein et al., 1995). Although Heller et al. (1994) found that differences in coresidence between Latinos and non-Latinos were no longer significant when controlling for SES and child age, other studies found that Latino caregivers are more likely to prefer these arrangements (Kraemer & Blacher, 2008; Magaña & Smith, 2006b; Milstein et al., 1995; Rueda, Monzo, Shapiro, Gomez, & Blacher, 2005). In a qualitative study, Rueda et al. (2005) found that the predominant theme among Latina mothers of children with ID was the belief that no one could care better for their child than themselves. In a study comparing non-Latina White mothers to Latina mothers who were coresiding with their youth and adults with autism, researchers found that Latina mothers were more satisfied with the living arrangement than the White mothers, which was related to lower levels of psychological distress and higher levels of psychological well-being among the Latina mothers (Magaña & Smith, 2006b).

RESEARCH ON OUT-OF-HOME PLACEMENT OF PERSONS WITH ID AND MENTAL ILLNESS

Factors that may precipitate placing a son or daughter with ID or mental illness outside the family home include high levels of maladaptive behaviors, severe physical impairments of the son or daughter, caregiver stress, and declining physical capacity of the caregiver (Heller & Factor, 1994; Seltzer et al., 1997). Seltzer et al. (1997) found differential factors predicting out-of-home placement for adults with IDs versus severe mental illness. Predictors for mothers caring for an adult with ID were older mothers' age and poorer health, and whether their child was on a waiting list for placement. On the other hand, gender of the person with mental illness, increased venting of emotions by the caregiver, and psychiatric crisis were predictors of out-of-home placement for caregivers of adults with mental illness. Another risk factor predicting out-of-home placement of children with ID includes reaching adolescence (Blacher & Hanneman, 1993). As physical maturation of the child increases, so do their daily needs (Blacher & Bromley, 1990). It is possible that similar factors may influence Latino family caregivers; however, due to a strong cultural commitment to live with the son or daughter they may have higher thresholds for these factors.

A few studies have explored the relationship between out-of-home placement and caregiver well-being for parents who have a son or a daughter with developmental disabilities or severe mental illnesses like schizophrenia. The majority of the studies focused on people with ID and found that parents who lived apart from their child reported more positive well-being outcomes compared to when they were living with their child (Baker & Blacher, 2002; Gallagher & Mechanic, 1996; Seltzer et al., 1997; Werner, Edwards, & Baum, 2009). For example, Baker and Blacher (2002) found that caregivers experienced reduced stress, increased peace of mind, and increased opportunities to pursue a career or personal interest. Gallagher and Mechanic (1996) found that caregivers reported better health and fewer physical limitations; and Warner et al. (2009) reported improved emotional well-being, social life and marital satisfaction, and overall quality of life. Investigating the role of end-of-coresidence on burden and depression among maternal caregivers of persons with ID and mental illness, Seltzer and colleagues (1997) found that end of coresidence predicted lower levels of subjective burden for mothers of adults with mental retardation as well as mothers of adults with mental illness; however, there was no difference in depressive symptoms. Only one study found no differences in any of the well-being outcomes examined between older caregivers of adults with ID who coreside with their son or daughter and those who do not coreside (McDermott, Valentine, Anderson, Gallup, & Thompson, 1997).

Interestingly, the gains or advantages identified by families following placement are also accompanied by ambivalent feelings of loss or guilt for having placed the child. The most common feeling is that of being unable to fulfill one's role as a parent (Baker & Blacher, 2002; Werner et al., 2009). However, much of this guilt and worry varies by the age of child being placed. As noted by Hayden and Heller (1997) and Baker and Blacher (2002), guilt and worry were characteristic of parents of young children. When compared to parents of adults with ID, parents of children with ID experienced high levels of burden, irrespective of their place of residence (Hayden & Heller). Similarly, families of children with ID when compared to others (families of adolescents, young adults, or adults) reported the lower levels of marital satisfaction and the higher levels of burden and stress. Thus, parents of young children with ID maybe more vulnerable to psychological distress when placing their child outside of the home (Baker & Blacher).

Overall, most research on placement and caregiver well-being provides evidence of better outcomes experienced by caregivers when their son or daughter with ID lives outside the home, particularly when their children are adults. However, this body of research has focused primarily on White caregiver samples. Thus more needs to be known about how Latina/o caregivers adapt to out-of-home placement.

CURRENT STUDY VARIABLES AND RESEARCH QUESTIONS

To determine what variables were important to include in our analyses, we took guidance from an article that discussed methodological challenges of research comparing families of children with autism with families of children with other disabilities (Seltzer, Abbeduto, Krauss, Greenberg, & Swe, 2004). The authors listed several variables for which adjustments are important. These variables include child or parent age, parent marital status, number of children in the family, child gender, time since diagnosis, and behavior problems as well as contextual variables such as parental education and ethnicity (Seltzer et al., 2004). Research on mothers of children with developmental disabilities find maternal health is important to take into account as well (Magaña, Seltzer, & Krauss, 2004). For Latinos, some form of acculturation is important to measure. A study of Cuban American mothers of adults with mental retardation found that greater levels of acculturation was related to lower levels of psychological distress (Magaña, Schwartz, Rubert, & Szapocznik, 2006).

Our research questions are exploratory as there is no clear evidence to suggest hypothesized relationships. Previous research summarized thus far suggests that though experiences may be different, well-being outcomes between mothers of children with autism and mothers of children schizophrenia may be very similar. Additionally, research that has focused on Latino caregiving has reported similar findings with respect to culture and family in individual studies despite different disability contexts. Our research questions are:

1. Do depressive symptoms and psychological well-being differ between Latina mothers of persons with autism and Latina mothers of persons with schizophrenia?
2. What are the most important predictors of depressive symptoms and psychological well-being for both groups of Latina caregiving mothers?
3. What is the relationship between mothers coresiding with their child and maternal outcomes, and are these relationships similar for both groups of mothers?

METHOD

Study Sample and Data Collection

Participants in the current analysis included Latina mothers from two separate but related studies designed to explore the experiences of caregiving families who have a son or a daughter with autism ($N = 29$) or schizophrenia ($N = 33$).

Latina mothers of children with autism were part of the first wave of a larger longitudinal study of aging mothers of adults or adolescents with a diagnosis of autism spectrum disorder (ASD) in Wisconsin and Massachusetts. The respondents for the current study were recruited through agencies, diagnostic clinics, and the media between 1998 and 2002. A special effort was made to recruit Latino families for the study, particularly in Massachusetts where more Latinos were connected to the service systems. The families in the Latino sample had three criteria that needed to be met for sample selection: (1) to have a son or a daughter 8 years old or older; (2) with a diagnosis of an ASD from a medical, psychological or educational professional, as reported by parents; and (3) a careful review of multiple sources of diagnostic information confirming the diagnosis for an ASD. The Autism Diagnostic

Interview-Revised (ADI-R), the Autism Behavior Checklist (ABC), and parental report were the primary sources of data used to ascertain diagnosis (Lord, Rutter, & Le Couteur, 1994; Krug, Arick, & Almond, 1980). There were 32 original mother–child dyads in the sample. However, because of missing data on the outcome variables we removed three cases. Therefore, the final sample size of mothers of children with autism was 29 in the current analyses. All interviews were conducted in the home of the participant.

Mothers of adults with schizophrenia were part of the first wave of a larger longitudinal study of aging families of adults with schizophrenia in Wisconsin. Criteria for inclusion in the study were that the respondent was the primary family caregiver of the person with schizophrenia, and the relative being cared for had a diagnosis of schizophrenia or schizoaffective disorder. To expand the number of Latino participants, recruitment was also conducted in Los Angeles, CA. There were 42 Latino caregivers in the study; however, 33 of them were the mothers of the person with schizophrenia (others were spouses, fathers, siblings, and other relatives), and only mothers were included in our current analyses (25 mothers from Los Angeles and 8 mothers from Wisconsin). The participants were recruited primarily through county mental health agencies, community support groups, and the media between 2000 and 2003. Caregivers were interviewed in their home or at the mental health agency, according to their preferences.

For both studies, interviews were conducted in the language of preference (Spanish or English) by bilingual and bicultural interviewers. All the instruments not already available in Spanish were translated using the translation/back-translation method (Kurtines & Szapocznik, 1995).

Measures

Dependent variables

Maternal psychological distress and well-being were the two dependent variables in the study. Psychological distress was measured by Radloff's (1977) Center for Epidemiological Studies Depression Scale (CES-D) and psychological well-being was measured by the sum of three subscales from Ryff's (1989) measure of psychological well-being. The CES-D is a valid and reliable measure of depressive symptoms in the general population, and its validity and reliability is also evident across cultural groups, including Latino population (Cho et al., 1993; Guarnaccia, Angel, & Worobey, 1989; Stroup-Benham, Lawrence, & Treviño, 1992). The CES-D consists of 20 items in which respondents report the frequency of depressive symptoms exhibited in the last week. For example, respondents are asked to indicate how often they felt unhappy, lonely, experienced crying spells, and had thoughts that life has been a failure etc., in the last one week. The measure uses a 4-point scale ranging from *rarely* = 0 (less than 1 day) to *most of the time* = 3

(5–7 days). Items were summed to obtain the total score. Possible scores range from 0 to 60, with higher scores indicating higher levels of depressive symptoms. The Cronbach's alpha for the present sample was .90.

A modified version of Ryff's (1989) psychological well-being measure was used to assess positive psychological well-being. Five items from each of three subscales (Personal Growth, Self Acceptance, and Purpose in Life) were used in both samples for a total of 15 items. Respondents rated their level of agreement for each item on a 6-point scale (1 = *strongly disagree* to 6 = *strongly agree*). Total score was calculated by summing their responses. Possible scores range from 15 to 90, with higher scores indicating positive psychological well-being. Respondents indicate the extent to which they are interested in activities that expand their horizon, feel positive with how life turned out to be, and that they have a sense of purpose and direction in life. Ryff's psychological well-being measure has been used successfully with Latino populations (Gloria, Castellanos & Orozco, 2005; Ryff, Keyes, & Hughes, 2004). Cronbach's alpha for the present sample was .82.

Maternal characteristics

Maternal characteristics were gathered in the demographic portion of the questionnaire and included age (in years), number of children in the family, marital status (1 = *married*, 0 = *not married*) level of education (1 = *less than high school*, 2 = *high school*, 3 = *some college*, 4 = *bachelor's degree or higher*), and total family income was calculated using a categorical variable where 1 indicated an annual income of $0 to $4,999, 2 indicated $5,000 to $9,999, and so on, to 13 indicated $70,000 and above. Although an acculturation scale was used in both studies, not all of the respondents received this part of the questionnaire. Therefore, to assess some level of acculturation, language of interview (0 = *English*, 1 = *Spanish*) was used as a proxy. Respondents were asked about their Latino ethnicity or country of origin. The two largest groups identified were Mexican/Mexican American and Puerto Rican. Other respondents were from the Caribbean (Dominican Republic and Cuba), Central America, and South America, but the numbers in each group were too small to statistically analyze. Therefore, we categorized Latino ethnicity as (1 = *Mexican*, 2 = *Puerto Rican*, and 3 = *Other Latino*).

Maternal health status was measured by a single item in which the mother rated her health on a 4 point scale (1 = *poor* to 4 = *excellent*), with higher score indicating better perceived health (Stewart, Hays, & Ware, 1988).

Youth/adult characteristics

Maladaptive behaviors were assessed through the Inventory for Client and Agency Planning (ICAP; Bruinicks, Hill, Weatherman, & Woodcock, 1986). The measure was adapted and validated for a Spanish-speaking population

(Montero, 1999). The ICAP is a measure of eight items that assesses the presence and severity of behavior problems across three domains: internalizing behaviors (behaviors being hurtful to one self), externalizing behaviors (behaviors hurtful to others), and asocial behaviors (socially uncooperative and offensive behavior). The respondents were asked to confirm the presence of a behavior problem and then report on the severity. The scale for maladaptive behavior problems was constructed by taking a count of the eight behavior problems reported as present. Possible scale values range from 0 to 8.

Other youth/adult characteristics included age (in years), place of residence (1 = *home*, 0 = *outside residence*), gender (0 = *son*, 1 = *daughter*), time since diagnosis (computed by subtracting year of diagnosis from year of interview), and health status based on mothers' report of son or daughters' health on a 4-point scale ranging from *poor* to *excellent*. The key youth/adult characteristic related to research question 1 is diagnosis (0 = *schizophrenia*, 1 = *ASD*).

Open-ended questions

We analyzed two open-ended questions that were asked of participants who were no longer coresiding with their son or daughter: (1) Could you describe for me why your (son or daughter) moved out of the home? (2) How do you feel about your (son or daughter) living outside the home?

Quantitative Data Analysis

In preliminary analyses, we examined differences between the two diagnostic groups on maternal and youth/adult characteristics using chi square and t test analyses. We also examined differences between the three Latino ethnicity groups on the dependent variables. After conducting a t test on dependent variables between the two diagnostic groups, ordinary least squares regression (OLS) was used to test our first research question. Hierarchical linear regression was used to test our second and third research questions. Regarding missing data, one mother (in the schizophrenia sample) did not fill out the Ryff Psychological Well-Being measure and was excluded from analyses involving this measure. Subsequently the N for the regressions using Ryff as a dependent measure was 61, while the N for the regressions using the CES-D was 62.

We conducted content analysis of two open-ended questions to further explore how mothers experienced living apart from their son or daughter. The procedure used in this analysis is outlined by Skinner, Rodriguez, and Bailey (1999) and included the following: First, the lead author and a graduate student reviewed the open-ended responses to the two questions on the nine cases in which mothers lived apart from their son or daughter to develop a tentative list of key themes. We then met to discuss and agree upon the themes that would be used for categorizing individual responses. We then reread the responses and categorized them into the themes that were developed. We met again to determine agreement with the decisions made.

RESULTS

Preliminary Analysis

Table 1 shows differences between the two diagnostic groups on maternal and youth/adult characteristics. Mothers of adults with schizophrenia were

TABLE 1 Maternal and Youth/Adult Characteristics

	Schizophrenia $N=33$	Autism N = 29	Test value (t or χ^2)
Maternal characteristics			
Age ($M \pm SD$)	59.8 (10.2)	44.1 (8.3)	6.5**
range	35–89	33–62	
# of children ($M \pm SD$)	2.4 (2.1)	1.7 (1.3)	1.8
Marital status (%)			
Married	51.5	27.6	3.7*
Annual income (percentage)			
\$0–19,999	57.0	65.5	2.4
\$20,000–39,999	18.2	20.7	
\$40,000–59,999	15.2	3.4	
\$60,000+	9.1	10.3	
Education (percentage)			
Less than high school	54.5	34.5	6.5
High school	15.2	31.0	
Some college	24.2	13.8	
Bachelor's and higher	6.1	20.7	
Health status (percentage)			
Excellent/good	48.5	51.7	.06
Language of interview (percentage)			
Spanish	81.8	65.5	2.1
Ethnicity (percentage)			
Mexican origin	42.4	0	17.9***
Puerto Rican	12.1	41.4	
Other Latino	45.5	58.6	
Youth/adult characteristics			
Age ($M \pm SD$)	36.3 (10.1)	16.7 (8.1)	8.5
range	19–65	8–40	
# of Maladaptive behaviors ($M \pm SD$)	1.8 (1.8)	3.6 (2.2)	−3.6***
Time since diagnosis	16.4 (9.5)	12.8 (8.0)	1.6
Residential status (percentage)			
Coresiding	87.9	82.8	0.3
placed	12.1	17.2	
Gender (percentage)			
Male	81.8	69.0	1.4
Health status (percentage)			
Good/excellent	42.4	79.3	8.7**

*$p < .05$, **$p < .01$, ***$p < .001$.

significantly older than mothers of youth/adults with autism. Mothers in the autism study were less likely to be married than mothers in the schizophrenia study. Although 14 (42.4%) mothers of adults with schizophrenia were of Mexican American descent, none of the mothers in the autism study was. About 12 (41.4%) mothers in the autism study were Puerto Rican whereas 4 (12.1%) mothers in the schizophrenia study mothers were. Health status, education, household income, and language of interviews did not differ between the two groups of mothers.

As expected, age of the person with a disability differed between the two groups, which was a function of recruitment criteria: the autism study recruited youth and adults from 8 years and older, whereas the schizophrenia study focused on adults. Other youth/adult characteristics that differed between the two diagnostic groups included behavior problems, those with autism had significantly higher levels, and physical health status, and persons with schizophrenia were in worse physical health. Gender, time since diagnosis, and residential status did not significantly differ between the two groups. More than 80% of offspring with autism ($N=24$) and schizophrenia ($N=29$) lived at home with their mothers.

An important preliminary question was to determine whether there were differences between mothers of Mexican, Puerto Rican, or other Latino descent in our dependent variables. We found that Mexican-descent mothers ($M=60.6$, $SD=12.9$) had significantly lower levels of psychological well-being than Puerto Rican mothers ($M=72.6$, $SD=12.9$) and other Latina mothers. $M=71.3$, $SD=10.3$, $F(2, 58)=5.0$, $p=.01$. Mothers of Puerto Rican and other Latino descent were not significantly different from each other on these two dependent variables. Because there are no mothers of Mexican descent in the autism sample, we also examined these differences within the schizophrenia sample to ensure the ethnicity differences we found were not a function of difference in diagnosis. We found that the means of the three ethnic groups within the schizophrenia group were very similar to those in our overall sample. Therefore, we created a dummy variable (0 = *other Latino*, 1 = *Mexican descent*) and used it in our subsequent analyses.

Research Question 1

In our first research question, we asked whether depressive symptoms and psychological well-being differed between mothers of youth and adults with autism and mothers of adults with schizophrenia. Bivariate comparisons indicated that there are no differences between the two groups on depressive symptoms; however, the mothers of the youth/adults with autism reported higher levels of psychological well-being (see Table 2). In our regression analyses shown on Tables 3 and 4, these findings remain consistent even while adjusting for other variables in the model; caring for a child with

TABLE 2 Mean-Level Differences of Depressive Symptoms and Psychological Well-Being

	Schizophrenia ($N=33^a$)		Autism ($N=29$)		
	M	*SD*	*M*	*SD*	*t* statistic
Depressive symptoms	15.0	11.7	13.2	11.6	.6
Psychological well-being	65.9	12.5	72.8	11.3	−2.3*

[a]32 mothers of adults with schizophrenia completed the psychological well-being measure.
*$p<.05$.

TABLE 3 Regression of Depressive Symptoms ($N=62$)

	Model 1			Model 2		
Predictors	b	*SE*	*β*	b	*SE*	*β*
Diagnosis	−6.25	4.19	−.27	−7.88	4.05	−.34
Behavior problems	1.55	.72	.29*	1.51	.68	.28*
Time since diagnosis	.06	.21	.47**	.59	.19	.46**
Age of mother	−.46	1.49	−.48*	−.54	.19	−.57**
Mothers health	−2.93	3.68	−.24	−3.41	1.44	−.27*
Ethnicity	4.21	3.22	.15	3.71	3.52	.14
Language of interview	5.68	.22	6.54	3.09	.25*	
Child's place of residence	9.42	3.74	.29*			
Adjusted R^2			21***		28***	

Note: Diagnosis (0 = schizophrenia, 1 = autism); Ethnicity (0 = others, 1 = Mexican descent); Language of interview (0 = English, 1 = Spanish); Residence (0 = co-residing, 1 = placed).
*$p<.05$, **$p<.01$, ***$p<.001$.

TABLE 4 Regression of Psychological Well-being ($N=61$)

	Model 1			Model 2		
Predictors	b	*SE*	*β*	b	*SE*	*β*
Diagnosis	11.34	4.22	.46*	12.55	4.15	.51**
Behavior problems	−1.38	72	−.24	−1.35	.70	.23
Time since diagnosis	−.63	.21	−.42**	−.63	.20	−.42**
Age of mother	.58	.20	.53**	.62	.20	.57**
Mothers health	.57	1.52	.04	.85	1.48	.06
Ethnicity	−8.11	3.72	−.28*	−7.45	3.64	−.26*
Language of interview	−7.03	3.26	−.25*	−7.98	3.21	−.29*
Child's place of residence				−7.91	3.98	−.22
Adjusted R2			.29***			.37***

Note: Diagnosis (0 = schizophrenia, 1 = autism); Ethnicity (0 = others, 1 = Mexican descent); Language of interview (0 = English, 1 = Spanish); Residence (0 = co-residing, 1 = placed).
*$p<.05$, **$p<.01$, ***$p<.001$.

schizophrenia predicts lower levels of psychological well-being but is not related to depressive symptoms.

Research Question 2

In our second research question we asked what the most important predictors were of depressive symptoms and psychological well-being for mothers of youth/adults with autism and schizophrenia. To answer this question, we conducted OLS regression. Because of our limited sample size, we needed to reduce the number of variables used in the regression models to maximize the degrees of freedom. First, we decided to use maternal age rather than son or daughter age because these variables are highly correlated with each other and because the focus of our analysis is on maternal outcomes. We then examined correlations of all independent variables (maternal and child characteristics) with the dependent variables; however, only one independent variable was statistically significant in bivariate correlations–level of education. Greater levels of education was related to greater levels of psychological well-being ($r = .31$, $p = .02$) and lower levels of depressive symptoms ($r = -.27$, $p = .04$). We then tested all of the maternal and child characteristics in regression models to determine their relationship to the dependent variables while adjusting for the others, and to determine multicollinearity effects with other variables in the model. Variables that did not contribute to the regression models were marital status, number of children, maternal education, income, sons or daughters' health and gender; therefore they were removed in the final models. We report regression analyses separately for the two dependent variables—depressive symptoms and psychological well-being.

Table 3 Model 1 shows that more behavior problems, a longer time since diagnosis, and younger maternal age were related to higher levels of depressive symptoms. This model explained 21% of the variance in maternal depression.

In addition to the relationship between caring for a child with schizophrenia and lower levels of psychological well-being, the following items were related to higher levels of psychological well-being: shorter time since diagnosis, older maternal age, not being of Mexican descent, and interviews conducted in English (see Table 4). Overall, the model explained 29% of the variance in maternal psychological well-being. Findings that were common across the two maternal outcomes were that mothers being younger and mothers experiencing a longer time since diagnosis predicted worse outcomes.

Research Question 3

We asked whether there was a relationship between coresiding with a child with autism or schizophrenia and the maternal outcomes in the current study.

Table 3 Model 2 shows that mothers who lived apart from their son or daughter had significantly higher levels of depressive symptoms. Furthermore, two of the variables that were not related in Model 1 became statistically significant: poorer maternal health and interview conducted in Spanish were related to higher depressive symptoms after taking into account whether the son or daughter was living at home. The explained variance in Model 2 for depressive symptoms was 28%.

Having a son or daughter who lived at home was not significantly related to greater levels of psychological well-being (see Table 4 Model 2); However, the p value was barely above the cut-off for statistical significance ($p = .052$). Consistent with Model 1, having a son or daughter with autism, shorter time since diagnosis, older maternal age, other Latino descent, and interview conducted in English were significantly related to greater levels of psychological well-being. Findings explained 37% of the variance in Model 2.

Open-Ended Analysis

In this analysis, we wished to explore open-ended data in the current study to better understand why having the son or daughter living outside the home might be contributing to higher levels of depressive symptoms among these mothers. There were a total of nine such cases in our sample, four from the schizophrenia study and five from the autism study.

Reasons for their son or daughter moving out of the home that emerged from this analysis were severe behavior problems, educational opportunities for the son or daughter, deteriorating caregiver health, and the decision of the son or daughter. Themes that emerged regarding how mothers felt about their son or daughter living apart included feeling like mothers could live a normal life, and feelings of deep sadness and guilt. These sentiments were often experienced simultaneously.

For all of the cases in the autism study (three males and two females age between 10 and 27 years), mothers reported severe behavior problems such as biting or hurting self and others, destroying property, and staying up all night as the reason for placement in a residential facility. Parents generally felt they were unable to manage behaviors and needed help. Two mothers also indicated that the placement was better for their son or daughter and would provide important education that they needed. Mothers reported some of the positive aspects of living apart from their son or daughter such as "living a normal life," spending more time with their other children, and attending church. However, great sadness was conveyed as well by all of the mothers. For example, one mother said,

> But my greatest wish is to be able to have her live with us. I miss her a lot. I wish to take care of her and give her a lot of a mother's love and that she

> lives with her family and tries to live a normal life. And I would like to give her everything she wants. Without my daughter I feel empty.

Another said,

> It is very difficult but I love my son and I always pray to God that I live a long life to take care of my son. I love him with all of my heart. If there is anything to change the way he is I would give my life for that.

A third mother put it succinctly by stating, "*Me hace mucha falta*" (I miss him very much).

Mothers of adults with schizophrenia had less choice in the matter of whether their son or daughter lived with them. All four of the cases were sons, and for three of those cases mothers indicated that their son chose to live on his own or elsewhere. In two cases, mothers cited extreme psychiatric conditions, or being up all night as reasons contributing to him living away from home. In another case, the son had moved from place to place due to behavioral issues such as getting into fights with other residents or coworkers, and was in jail at the time of the interview. This mother had been through a lifetime of traumas and what she referred to as a dysfunctional family. She reported that another son had committed suicide many years before, and her other children were addicted to drugs or not functioning well. She felt that she was unable to help her children and stated that she was in a lot of emotional pain due to being at her limit, disoriented, and impotent to help. Another mother indicated that her heart problems coupled with her son's behavioral issues prompted her to seek outside placement. This mother said, "I have chosen to detach myself from his daily care because of the tremendous impact it has had on my health and my depression as a result of his problems." One mother who was a widow wanted her son to come home, but psychiatrists did not recommend it. She felt guilty, sad, and stressed about his living situation.

DISCUSSION

The current study focused on two unique caregiving experiences among Latina mothers: that of caring for a youth or adult with autism and that of caring for an adult with schizophrenia. One of the main differences between the two groups of care recipients besides age was that the son or daughter with autism had higher levels of behavior problems than the son or daughter with schizophrenia. Also, the adults with schizophrenia, who were on average older, were in worse physical health than the persons with autism. Mothers of the adults with schizophrenia were older and more likely to be married than mothers of youth or adults with autism.

Our analyses showed that mothers of youth or adults with autism had higher levels of psychological well-being than mothers of adults with schizophrenia. This finding is unique as previous research that has used the same psychological well-being measure found no differences between White mothers of adults with autism and schizophrenia (Greenberg et al., 2004). The mean levels of psychological well-being of the Latina mothers caring for a child with autism were similar to the levels reported in the Greenberg et al. (2004) study whereas the mean levels for Latina mothers in the current schizophrenia sample were much lower. Although there was no significant difference in the years since diagnosis for both groups of mothers in the current study, the experiences of adapting to the diagnosis and feeling positive about it may differ. Our measure of psychological well-being consisted of three subscales: Personal Growth, Self-Acceptance, and Purpose in Life (Ryff, 1989). Because parents learn about autism early in the child's life, they may be more accepting of the child as someone special in their lives that can contribute to their purpose in life, accepting of themselves, and feeling like they have grown personally. In contrast, parents learn about schizophrenia later in their child's life when things may have been going well from the parents' perspective but are suddenly interrupted by their young adult child exhibiting strange behaviors and activities. For Latino parents of adults with schizophrenia who are more likely than White parents to live with their child and see them suffer on a daily basis, their personal outlook on their own life may be less positive.

We did not find significant differences between the two groups of mothers in levels of depressive symptoms. As reported in other studies, we found that higher levels of care recipient behavior problems and poorer maternal health (when controlling for child's place of residence) were related to higher levels of maternal depressive symptoms across disability groups (Abbeduto et al., 2004; Pruchno & Patrick, 1999; Magaña, Seltzer, & Krauss, 2004). Similar findings in other studies have been robust across disability and ethnic groups. For this reason, services and treatments that work to reduce behavioral problems among persons with autism and mental illness would benefit parental caregivers in addition to the person with the disability. Some of these may include psychoeducational models that show parents how to respond to maladaptive behaviors or psychiatric symptoms (Cohen et al., 2008; McIntyre, 2008). These services are mostly used for caregivers of persons with serious mental illness but may be emerging in the autism field. Services of psychologists or behaviorists who can provide consultations to parents and treatment for the person with the disability and that are culturally and linguistically appropriate may serve to reduce maladaptive behaviors and subsequently depressive symptoms in Latina mothers.

At the same time it is important to note that the relationship of maladaptive behaviors and maternal depressive symptoms can have bidirectional effects in which behaviors predict more depressive symptoms overtime, but depressive symptoms can also predict higher levels of maladaptive behaviors overtime (Orsmond, Seltzer, Krauss, & Hong, 2003). Because some research has found that mothers of offspring with schizophrenia and autism are more likely to have psychological problems (Daniels et al., 2008; Faridi, Pawliuk, King, Joober, & Malla, 2009), attention and resources should be given to the treatment of psychological distress in mothers as much in treating behavior problems in the son or daughter.

An interesting finding for both maternal outcomes in the current study was that older maternal age was related to better outcomes, a finding that is consistent with research on Latina mothers of adults with schizophrenia and ID (Magaña et al., 2007; Magaña & Smith, 2006a). Although maternal age significantly correlates with time since diagnosis as would be expected, time since diagnosis is related to higher levels of depressive symptoms and lower levels of psychological well-being when adjusting for maternal age and other factors, thus demonstrating the independent contribution of each of these variables. This finding that suggests that the accumulation of time caring for a person with either disorder may take its toll on Latina mothers. At the same time older mothers may have learned effective coping strategies over the course of their child's illness.

Other interesting relationships we found in the current study were that mothers of Mexican descent had lower levels of psychological well-being than other Latina mothers, and mothers who were primarily Spanish speaking had higher levels of depressive symptoms and lower levels of psychological well-being in our final models. Because all of the mothers of Mexican descent were mothers of adults with schizophrenia, it is difficult to tease out whether the former relationship is due to the schizophrenia caregiving or a cultural factor related to being of Mexican descent. Using language of interview as a rough proxy for acculturation, the latter finding suggests that more acculturated mothers may have better well-being outcomes than less acculturated mothers. This finding is consistent with previous research of Latino parents of adults with developmental disabilities and may be due in part to stressors mothers face in navigating the service and treatment systems that are primarily English based for their son or daughter (Magaña et al., 2006).

Our finding related to our last research question was that mothers whose son or daughter was living outside the home had higher levels of depressive symptoms. More than 80% of the mothers in both studies lived with their son or daughter which is quite remarkable in itself. There were nine mothers who did not live with their son or daughter, and we explored their experiences more in-depth. What emerged in the open-ended data was that for mothers of children with autism, a placement decision was typically made because of extreme behavioral issues that parents were unable to handle. Although mothers in these cases were able to talk about things that were better in their lives, they expressed a profound sadness about not being able to provide their child with the family and caring experiences they thought he or she deserved. Baker and Blacher (2002) found similar results for non-Latina mothers of young children with ID; however, they found that mothers of adults with ID had better outcomes. The children in our sample were not young children; however, two of the children with autism that lived outside the home were younger than age 18 (ages 10 and 13), and the other three were adults. Mothers of adults with schizophrenia had less say about whether their sons moved out (all of the cases were male). However, they also cited behavioral concerns as well as their own health as factors that contributed to their son moving out. Consistent with other research on out-of-home placement, mothers from both groups described feelings of guilt for having to live apart from their son or daughter, and in some cases these feelings were experienced simultaneously with the positive feelings (Baker & Blacher). What is unique about our findings is that Latino caregivers of adults and older children with disabilities had worse outcomes if their child lived outside the home; whereas most research on non-Latino caregivers of adults has found the opposite (Baker & Blacher, 2002; Gallagher & Mechanic, 1996; Seltzer et al., 1997; Werner et al., 2009).

There are a few limitations to the current study. We used a convenient sample with a small number of Latino families that limits generalizability of the findings to all Latino families caring for a son or a daughter with autism or schizophrenia and limits the detection of significant relationships. Another limitation is that there were no Latinos of Mexican descent in our autism sample, which made it difficult to determine differences between Latino ethnicities. Participants in the current study volunteered to participate that increased the likelihood that our sample includes only those who were most willing to share information and had time to participate in a research study. The participants were primarily recruited through service agencies, and it is difficult to say whether families who are not in the system face more or fewer challenges. It is not known how recruitment from different sampling sites may have influenced the findings in the current study. Differences in services vary for autism and schizophrenia from one state to the other, and it is not known whether services have an impact on the well-being of caregiving Latinas. Last, the cross-sectional nature of the study limited our ability to detect the direction of relationship between variables.

Implications for future research suggest that a larger longitudinal study of caregivers of adults with autism and adults of schizophrenia would be able to confirm or negate findings and explore trends found in the current study. To control for the limitations from the current study, the larger study could be multisite, but would need to include persons with autism and persons with schizophrenia from the same cities, and ensure that major Latino ethnicities are represented in both disability groups. Future research should also examine similar well-being outcomes among Latino adults with schizophrenia and

Latinos adults with autism to determine how they experience living at home versus in an out-of-home setting.

Despite the small sample size, the current study found a number of significant relationships that have implications for practice. The current study sensitizes us to the unique cultural context within which Latina mothers of children with autism and schizophrenia provide care. The predominant goal of services for individuals with autism or schizophrenia is focused on independent living, which may not be appropriate for all ethnic communities. Caring for the person well into adulthood with autism or schizophrenia in the home may be culturally appropriate for Latino families. Therefore service systems need to address the special needs of parents who would like to care for their children at home, as well as modify goals and objectives of treatment to adapt to the cultural context of caregivers.

On the other hand, the current study suggests that there are circumstances, such as extreme and difficult behaviors as well as declining health of the parental caregiver, in which Latino families must resort to having their child live outside the home. Due to cultural pressures, mothers may feel guilty resorting to this decision and may need help and validation within the context of their cultural values to accept this decision. For example, helping the mother to consider the well-being of the whole family and how the family may benefit from increased attention to their needs, to continue to provide care to their son or daughter by visiting and making phone calls if they desire, and involving other family members in overseeing the son or daughter's care in the outside residence may help maternal caregivers accept their decision as a good one.

Another important issue for practice with Latino family caregivers is the finding that Spanish speaking Latina mothers had poorer well-being compared to the English speaking counterparts. This finding suggests that language barriers may make it difficult to navigate service delivery systems. Therefore, agencies need to have bilingual and bicultural service coordinators that can communicate with and adequately assess the needs of Spanish speaking families.

Service agencies must try to address the needs of caregivers over time, because the current study found a relationship between higher depressive symptoms, lower levels of psychological well-being, and time since diagnosis. This may arise due to parents having lower expectations for recovery for a child with a disability, as well as increasing concern over the future of the child. There may be different needs that caregivers have at different stages of the life course of caring for their son or daughter.

Finally, as discussed earlier, the strong relationship of behavior problems to depressive symptoms found in the current study indicates the need to address treatment of the behavior problems of the son or daughter and treatment of psychological distress among mothers in a culturally and linguistically relevant manner utilizing a two-pronged approach.

REFERENCES

Abbeduto, L., Seltzer, M. M., Shattuck, P. T., Krauss, M. K., Orsmond, G. I., & Murphy, M. M. (2004). Psychological well-being and coping in mothers of youths with autism, Down syndrome, of fragile X syndrome. *Journal on Mental Retardation, 9*(103), 237–254.

American Psychiatric Association. (2000). *Diagnostic and statistical manual of mental disorders* (4th ed.). Washington, DC: Author.

Aranda, M. P., & Knight, B. G. (1997). The influence of ethnicity and culture on the caregiver stress and coping process: A sociocultural review and analysis. *The Gerontologist, 37*, 342–354.

Baker, B. L., & Blacher, J. (2002). For better or worse? Impact of residential placement on families. *Mental Retardation, 40*, 1–13.

Blacher, J., & Bromley, B. (1990). Factors influencing and factors preventing placement of severely handicapped children: Perspectives from mothers and fathers. In W. I. Fraser (Ed.), *Key issues in mental retardation research* (pp. 222–235). London: Routledge.

Blacher, J., & Hanneman, R. (1993). Out-of-home placement of children and adolescents with severe handicaps: Behavioral intentions and behavior. *Research in Developmental Disabilities, 14*, 145–160.

Blacher, J., Lopez, S., Shapiro, J., & Fusco, J. (1997). Contributions to depression in Latina mothers with and without children with retardation: Implications for caregiving. *Family Relations, 46*, 325–334.

Bruininks, R. H., Hill, B. K., Weatherman, R. F., & Woodcock, R. W. (1986). *Inventory for client and agency planning*. Allen, TX: DLM Teaching Resources.

Cho, M. J., Mocícki, E. K., Narrow, W. E., Rae, D. S., Locke, B. Z., & Regier, D. A. (1993). Concordance between two measures of depression in the Hispanic Health and Nutrition Exam Survey. *Social Psychiatry and Psychiatric Epidemiology, 28*, 156–163.

Cohen, A. N., Glynn, S. M., Murray-Swank, A. B., Barrio, C., Fischer, E. P., McCutcheon, S. J., et al. (2008). The family forum: Directions for the implementation of family psychoeducation for severe mental illness. *Psychiatric Services, 59*, 40–48.

Cohn, D. (2003, June 19). Hispanics declared largest minority: Blacks overtaken in census update. *The Washington Post*, p. A1.

Daniels, J., Forssen, U., Hultman, C., Cnattingius, S., Savitz, D., Feychting, M., et al. (2008). Parental psychiatric disorders associated with autism spectrum disorders in offspring. *Pediatrics, 121*, e1357–e1362.

Faridi, K., Pawliuk, N., King, S., Joober, R., & Malla, A. (2009). Prevalence of psychotic and non-psychotic disorders in relatives of patients with a first episode psychosis. *Schizophrenia Research, 114*, 57–63.

Gallagher, S. K., & Mechanic, D. (1996). Living with the mentally ill: Effects on the health and functioning of other household members. *Social Science and Medicine, 42*, 1691–1701.

Gloria, A., Castellanos, J., & Orozco, V. (2005). Perceived educational barriers, cultural fit, coping responses and psychological well-being of Latina undergraduates. *Hispanic Journal of Behavioral Sciences, 27*, 161–183.

Greenberg, J. S., Seltzer, M. M., & Greenley, J. R. (1993). Aging parents of adults with disabilities: The gratifications and frustrations of later life caregiving. *The Gerontologist, 33*, 542–550.

Greenberg, J. S., Seltzer, M. M., Krauss, M. W., Chou, R. J. A., & Hong, J. (2004). The effect of quality of the relationship between mothers and adult children with schizophrenia, autism, or Down syndrome on maternal well-being: The mediating role of optimism. *American Journal of Orthopsychiatry, 74*, 14–25.

Guarnaccia, P. J., Angel, R., & Worobey, J. L. (1989). The factor structure of the CES-D in the Hispanic Health and Nutrition Examination Survey: The influences of ethnicity, gender and language. *Social Science & Medicine, 29*, 85–94.

Guarnaccia, P. J., & Parra, P. (1996). Ethnicity, social status, and families' experiences of caring for a mentally ill family member. *Community Mental Health Journal, 32*, 243–260.

Hayden, M. F., & Heller, T. (1997). Support, problem-solving/coping ability, and personal burden of younger and older caregivers of adults with mental retardation. *Mental Retardation, 35*, 364–372.

Heller, T., & Factor, A. (1994). Facilitating future planning and transitions out of the home. In M. M. Seltzer, M. W. Krauss, & M. P. Janicki (Eds.), *Life course perspectives on adulthood and old age* (pp. 39–52). Washington, DC: American Association on Mental Retardation.

Heller, T., Markwardt, R., Rowitz, L., & Farber, B. (1994). Adaptation of Hispanic families to a member with mental retardation. *American Journal of Mental Retardation, 99*, 289–300.

Kraemer, B. R., & Blacher, J. (2008). Transition for Hispanic and Anglo young adults with severe intellectual disability: Parent perspectives over time. *Journal of Developmental Disabilities, 14*, 59–72.

Krug, D. A., Arick, J. R., & Almond, P. J. (1980). Behavior checklist for identifying severely handicapped individuals with high levels of autistic behavior. *Journal of Child Psychology and Psychiatry, 21*, 221–229.

Kurtines, W. M., & Szapocznik, J. (1995). Cultural competence in assessing Hispanic youths and families: Challenges in the assessment of treatment needs and treatment evaluation for Hispanic drug-abusing adolescents. *NIDA Research Monograph, 156*, 172–189.

Lord, C., Rutter, M., & Le Couteur, A. (1994). Autism diagnostic interview-revised: A revised version of a diagnostic interview for caregivers of individuals with possible pervasive developmental disorders. *Journal of Autism and Developmental Disorders, 24*, 659–685.

Magaña, S. (1999). Puerto Rican families caring for an adult with mental retardation: The role of familism. *American Journal on Mental Retardation, 104*, 466–482.

Magaña, S. (2006). Older Latino family caregivers. In B. Berkman (Ed.), *Handbook of social work in health and aging* (pp. 371–380). New York: Oxford University Press.

Magaña, S. M., García, J. I. R., Hernández, M. G., & Cortez, R. (2007). Psychological distress among Latino family caregivers of adults with schizophrenia: The roles of burden and stigma. *Psychiatric Services, 58*, 378–384.

Magaña, S., Greenberg, J., & Seltzer, M. (2004). The health and well-being of Black mothers who care for their adult children with schizophrenia. *Psychiatric Services, 55*, 711–713.

Magaña, S., Schwartz, S. J., Rubert, M. P., & Szapocznik, J. (2006). Hispanic caregivers of adults with mental retardation: The importance of family functioning. *American Journal on Mental Retardation, 111*, 250–262.

Magaña, S., Seltzer, M. M., & Krauss, M. W. (2004). Cultural context of caregiving: Differences in depression between Puerto Rican and Non-Latina White mothers of adults with mental retardation. *Mental Retardation, 42*, 1–11.

Magaña, S., & Smith, M. J. (2006a). Health outcomes of midlife and older Latina and Black American mothers of children with developmental disabilities. *Mental Retardation, 44*, 224–234.

Magaña, S., & Smith, M. J. (2006b). Psychological distress and well-being of Latina and Non-Latina White Mothers of youth and adults with an autism spectrum disorder: Cultural attitudes towards co-residence status. *American Journal of Orthopsychiatry, 76*, 346–357.

McDermott, S., Valentine, D., Anderson, D., Gallup, D., & Thompson, S. (1997). Parents of adults with mental retardation living in-home and out-of-home: Caregiving burdens and gratifications. *American Journal of Orthopsychiatry, 67*, 323–329.

McIntyre, L. L. (2008). Parent training for young children with developmental disabilities: Randomized controlled trial. *American Journal on Mental Retardation, 113*, 356–368.

Milstein, G., Guarnaccia, P., & Midlarsky, E. (1995). Ethnic differences in the interpretation of mental illness: Perspectives of caregivers. *Research in Community and Mental Health, 8*, 155–178.

Montero, D. (1999). *Educación de la conducta adaptativa en personas con discapacidades. Adaptación y validación del ICAP* [Evaluation of adaptive behavior of persons with disabilities: Adaptation and evaluation of the ICAP]. Bilbao: Instituto de Ciencias de la Educación, Universidad de Deusto (Tercera edición en Bilbao: Ediciones Mensajero, 1999). [Evaluation of adaptive behavior of persons with disabilities: Adaptation and evaluation of the ICAP. Bilbao: Institute of science in education, Deusto University (third edition in Balbao: Messenger Edition, 1999)].

Orsmond, G., Seltzer, M. M., Krauss, M. W., & Hong, J. (2003). Behavioral problems in adults with mental retardation and maternal well-being: Examination of direction of effects. *American Journal on Mental Retardation, 108*, 257–271.

Pruchno, R., & Patrick, J. (1999). Mothers and fathers of adults with chronic disabilities. *Research on Aging, 21*(5), 682–714.

Radloff, L. S. (1977). The CES-D Scale: A self-report depression scale for research in the general population. *Applied Psychological Measurement, 1*, 385–401.

Rueda, R., Monzo, L., Shapiro, J., Gomez, J., & Blacher, J. (2005). Cultural models of transition: Latina mothers of young adults with developmental disabilities. *Exceptional Children, 71*, 401–414.

Ryff, C. D. (1989). Happiness is everything, or is it? Explorations on the meaning of psychological well-being. *Journal of Personality and Social Psychology, 57*, 1069–1081.

Ryff, C. D., Keyes, C. L., & Hughes, D. L. (2004). Psychological wellbeing in MIDUS: Profiles of racial, ethnic diversity and life course uniformity. In O. G. Brim, C. D. Ryff, & R. C. Kessler (Eds.), *How healthy are we? A national study of well-being at midlife* (pp. 398–422). Chicago: University of Chicago Press.

Seltzer, M. M., Abbeduto, L., Krauss, M. W., Greenberg, J., & Swe, A. (2004). Comparison groups in autism family research: Down syndrome, fragile X syndrome, and schizophrenia. *Journal of Autism and Developmental Disorders*, *34*, 41–48.

Seltzer, M. M., Greenberg, J. S., Floyd, F. J., & Hong, J. (2004). Accommodative coping and well-being of midlife parents of children with mental health problems or developmental disabilities. *American Journal of Orthopsychiatry*, *74*, 87–195.

Seltzer, M. M., Greenberg, J. S., Floyd, F. J., Pettee, Y., & Hong, J. (2001). Life-course impacts of parenting a child with a disability. *American Journal on Mental Retardation*, *106*, 265–286.

Seltzer, M. M., Greenberg, J. S., Krauss, M. W., & Hong, J. (1997). Predictors and outcomes of the end of co-resident caregiving in aging families of adults with mental retardation or mental illness. *Family Relations*, *46*, 13–22.

Shattuck, P. T., Seltzer, M. M., Greenberg, J. S., Orsmond, G. I., Bolt, D., Kring, S., et al. (2007). Change in autism symptoms and maladaptive behaviors in adolescents and adults with an autism spectrum disorder. *Journal of Autism and Developmental Disorders*, *37*, 1735–1747.

Skinner, D., Rodriguez, P., & Bailey, D. B. Jr. (1999). Qualitative analysis of Latino parents' religious interpretations of their child's disability. *Journal of Early Intervention*, *22*, 271–285.

Stewart, A. L., Hays, R. D., & Ware, J. E. Jr. (1988). The MOS Short-Form General Health Survey: Reliability and validity in a patient population. *Medical Care*, *26*, 724–735.

Stroup-Benham, C. A., Lawrence, R. H., & Treviño, F. M. (1992). CES-D factor structure among Mexican American and Puerto Rican women from single- and couple-headed households. *Hispanic Journal of Behavioral Sciences*, *14*, 310–326.

Werner, S., Edwards, M., & Baum, N. T. (2009). Family quality of life before and after out-of-home placement of a family member with an intellectual disability. *Journal of Policy and Practice in Intellectual Disabilities*, *6*, 32–39.

Family Quality of Life: A Framework for Policy and Social Service Provisions to Support Families of Children With Disabilities

MIAN WANG

Gevirtz Graduate School of Education, University of California, Santa Barbara, California

ROY BROWN

School of Child and Youth Care, University of Victoria, Canada

As a new extension of individual quality-of-life (QOL) framework that has been widely embraced in the field of disability to affect policy making, guide service delivery, and enhance outcomes of individuals with disabilities, family quality of life (FQoL) has been increasingly recognized as an important concept in the area of family supports for families of children with disabilities in the last two decades. This article provides an overview of FQoL conceptualization by introducing two conceptual frameworks that are influential in the international research literature of FQoL and individuals with intellectual and developmental disabilities. In addition to the delineation of conceptualization and measurement development of FQoL, the article addresses issues of FQoL applications to professions such as social work and special education. Implications for policy, research, and practice with respect to family support for families of children with disabilities are also discussed.

Family quality of life (FQoL), as a natural extension of quality-of-life (QOL) research for individuals with intellectual and developmental disabilities, has emerged in the last decade as an important concept to influence policy making, guide service delivery, and enhance outcomes of individuals with disabilities and their families (Brown & Brown, 2004; Turnbull, Brown, & Turnbull, 2004). Research on FQoL, albeit in its infancy, has its roots in the related QOL, which focuses on the individual rather than the family. In the field of intellectual and developmental disabilities, the conceptualization of QOL for individuals with disabilities has gradually matured over the last 30 years (Brown, 1997; Cummins, 1997a; Felce, 1997; Goode, 1994; Schalock, 2000). Many QOL definitions have been put forward in the international literature (Hughes and Hwang, 1996). However, most seem to contain similar major ideas: (a) a life of quality is based on individual needs, choices, and control and is experienced when his or her needs are met and when he or she has the opportunity to pursue life enrichment in major life environments across the life span (Brown & Brown, 2003); and (b) QOL, including both subjective and objective aspects, is a multidimensional construct consisting of personal and environmental factors (Schalock, Brown, Brown, et al., 2002). The QOL conceptual framework and its key principles have provided a solid foundation for the rapid growth of FQoL research and have significantly impacted and shaped the emerging work on FQoL.

The field of social work has recognized the importance of QOL as a concept. It is noted that, as an ultimate goal of social service, the concept of QOL has been embraced in the mission statement of major international and national social work organizations (e.g., International Federation of Social Workers, National Association of Social Workers, Canadian Association of Social Workers) and included in a set of professional standards for different types of social workers promulgated by the National Association of Social Workers (NASW; NASW, 2002, 2003, 2005).

However, empirical studies on FQoL and application issues related to social work appear minimal. Through a brief literature search in the major social work–related databases such as Social Science Abstracts, Social Work Abstracts, PsychINFO, and Social Service Abstracts, we found that only a few studies were related to the concept of QOL regarding families. These studies focused on understanding QOL of African American families who lived in a predominant White neighborhoods (Gettys, 1980); perceived QOL of families who adopted special needs children (Sar, 1994); effects of using day care services for older persons on FQoL (Gitlin, Reever, Dennis, Mathieu, & Hauck, 2006); effects of vacations on the QOL of caregivers (Mactavish, MacKay, & Iwasaki, 2007); QOL of single-parent families (Ihinger-Tallman, 1995; Nandi & Harris, 1999); and QOL of older family members (Evandrou & Glaser, 2004; Kutner, Mistretta, & Barnhart, 1999; Lowenstein, 2007; Teno, Mor, & Ward, 2005).

The lack of QOL research in the context of family life where there are children with intellectual and developmental disabilities is even more evident in the field of social work. The literature search aforementioned yielded no studies that focused on or were involved in the concept of FQoL. Therefore, it is necessary and imperative for the FQoL concept to be introduced to and promoted in the field of social work because it is the ultimate goal and valued outcome of policies and social services for individuals and their families. FQoL provides not only a framework for social services that aims to supporting individuals and their families but also a way for professionals to think about and work toward what brings satisfaction and joy to families that they serve.

In this article, we provide an overview of conceptualization, measurement, and application of FQoL; delineate how this important concept has been increasingly recognized by policy makers, researchers, and practitioners in the context of family supports for families of children with intellectual and developmental disabilities; and discuss policy, research, and practice implications for the field of social work.

QUALITY OF LIFE RESEARCH AND EVOLUTION OF FAMILY QUALITY OF LIFE

The trend of increasing recognition and application of the QOL framework in the disability field reflects a changing vision of and common language for the social movements, where the purpose of education, intervention, support, and services was to make life better for individuals with disabilities (Schalock, 2000). The QOL conceptualization, as expounded by Schalock and colleagues (2002), is based on an array of research from a variety of countries. One of the earliest studies looked at the development and behavior of persons with intellectual disabilities over a six-year period through assessments by their parents on the QOL issues of their child with a disability (Brown, Bayer, & Brown, 1992; Brown, Bayer & Macfarlane, 1989). Gradually this and other work was pulled together in several edited volumes (Brown, 1997; Goode, 1994; Renwick, Brown & Nagler, 1996). Despite the multitude of QOL conceptualizations by researchers with different perspectives and from different disciplines (Hughes & Hwang, 1996), a consensus has been reached among an international team of researchers on the key components of QOL conceptualization (Schalock, Brown, et al., 2002). Some of the key concepts and principles regarding QOL include values, lifespan, holism, self-image, choice, personal control, empowerment, rights, and antidiscrimination. Although the functional areas of QOL may be labeled differently, most agree that the common QOL domains are physical well-being, material well-being, social well-being, and emotional and productive well-being.

Furthermore, Schalock, Brown, et al. (2002) suggested that QOL is a multidimensional construct that consists of eight important domains: Emotional Well-being, Interpersonal Relationships, Material Well-being, Personal Development, Physical Well-being, Self-determination, Social

Inclusion, and Rights. Similarly, Brown and Brown (2003) pointed out that QOL includes social well-being, objective and subjective (perceptual) aspects of life, multidimensional aspects of life including friendship and family, meeting of basic needs and ability to achieve personal goals, and a person's desired conditions of living.

Brown and Brown (2003) also noted that the QOL concept should then be applied to practice and published a text to illustrate how, through research, application and professional practice. They explained how this was not only possible but also was now being applied in a number of services; they also recognized that practice and policy need to go hand in hand; without such links, QOL practice would fail due to bureaucratic and other conflicting requirements. They then went on to illustrate how, in practice, these concepts could be applied to families. This last aspect was further developed in collaborative work between a variety of researchers and applied professionals (see Turnbull et al., 2004).

In addition to the conceptualization of QOL, efforts also have been put forth on the development of QOL measures to assess QOL of individuals with disabilities and/or chronic illness since 1990s. Chief among these measures are the Comprehensive Quality of Life Scale (Cummins, 1997b), Quality of Life Indicators (Raphael, Renwick, & Brown, 1997), the Quality of Life Questionnaire (Schalock & Keith, 1993), the World Health Organization Quality of Life Assessment (WHOQOL; Group, 1998), and Cross-Cultural Survey of Quality of Life Indicators (Verdugo & Schalock, 2003). In addition, measurement of individual QOL was developed for individuals with different characteristics: individuals without disabilities (Andrews & Ben-Arieh, 1999; Arad, 2001; Chipuer, Bramston, & Pretty, 2003; Meuleners, Lee, Binns, & Lower, 2003), individuals with mental health challenges (Hansson, 2002), and individuals from culturally and linguistically diverse backgrounds (Blake & Anderson, 2000; Holloway & Carson, 2002).

POLICY CONTEXT OF FAMILY QUALITY OF LIFE

In 2003, The Arc of the United States, in collaboration with 40 other organizations (including the National Institute on Child Health and Human Development, Administration on Developmental Disabilities, Office of Special Education and Rehabilitation Services, and the President's Council on Mental Retardation), sponsored a national conference to articulate the policy promises the United States has made to its citizens with intellectual disabilities and their families. Approximately 250 participants who represented self-advocates, families of individuals with intellectual disabilities, service providers, researchers, and policy leaders met in 12 topical groups to address policy goals, the current knowledge base, recommendations for future research, and recommendations for the translation of research into practice.

One of the groups focused on family life. The participants in the topical group on family life worked collaboratively during the conference and over a subsequent nine-month period to articulate national goals, review the research literature, and prepare a chapter for a forthcoming book of conference proceedings. The work of the topical group on family life defines the policy context for FQoL as a research priority.

The participants defined families to include people who think of themselves as part of a family, whether or not they are related by blood or marriage, and who support and care for each other on a regular basis (Poston et al., 2003). They contextualized their deliberations of policy goals in the current knowledge base within the perspectives of family-systems theory (Turnbull & Turnbull, 2001a; Whitechurch & Constantine, 1993); life span considerations (Carter & McGoldrick, 1989; Rodgers & White, 1993; Turnbull & Turnbull, 2001b); and cultural and linguistic diversity, particularly as manifested in the intellectual disabilities field (Deardorff & Hollman, 1997; Fujiura & Yamaki, 2000; National Research Council, 2002; see Table 1).

In defining the policy context of family research goals, the group first reviewed Supreme Court decisions that underscore the family as the traditional core unit of American society (Troxel v. Granville, 2000; Wisconsin v. Yoder, 1972; see Table 2). These cases provide the policy context for the legal principle of "family as foundation" of American society (Turnbull, Beegle, & Stowe, 2001). The common law doctrine of *parens patriae* enables the government to limit state intervention into the family's traditional roles and to enhance the family's QOL. The group also conducted a policy analysis of Congressional statutes and Supreme Court decisions in order to identify a single overarching policy goal and other associated goals that reflect the country's "promises" to individuals with intellectual disabilities and their families pertaining specifically to family life (Turnbull et al., 2005).

TABLE 1 Family Life Goals Based on U.S. Policy

Overarching goal: To support the caregiving efforts and enhance the quality of life of all families so that families will remain the core unit of American society.

Goal 1: To ensure family–professional partnerships in research, policy making, and the planning and delivery of supports and services so that families will control their own destinies with due regard to the autonomy of adult family members with disabilities to control their own lives.

Goal 2: To ensure that families fully participate in communities of their choice through comprehensive, inclusive, neighborhood-based, and culturally responsive supports and services.

Goal 3: To ensure that services and supports for all families are available, accessible, appropriate, affordable, and accountable.

Goal 4: To ensure that sufficient public and private funding will be available to implement these goals and that all families will participate in directing the use of public funds authorized and appropriated for their benefits.

Goal 5: To ensure that families and professionals have full access to state-of-the-art knowledge and best practices and that they will collaborate in using knowledge and practices.

TABLE 2 Congressional Statutes and Supreme Court Cases Undergirding Family Goals

Individuals with Disabilities Education Act	Technical Assistance Act
Family Education Rights and Privacy Act	Adoption Assistance and Child Welfare Act
Developmental Disabilities Act	Child Abuse Prevention and Treatment Act
Title V, Social Security	Americans with Disabilities Act (1990)
Title XVI, Social Security	Rehabilitation Act (1973)
Title XVIII, Social Security	*Meyer V. Neb.* (1923)
Title XIX, Social Security	*Pierce v. Society of Sisters* (1925)
Title XX, Social Security	*Prince v. Mass.* (1944)
Title XXI, Social Security	*Stanley v. Ill.* (1972)
Katie Beckett	*Wisconsin v. Yoder* (1972)
Child Health Act	*Quilloin v. Walcott* (1978)
Health Insurance Portability and Accountability Act	*Parham v. J.R.* (1979)
Emergency Medical Treatment and Active Labor Act	*Santosky v. Kramer* (1982)
Family and Medical Leave Act	*Mississippi Band v. Holyfield* (1989)
Indian Child Welfare Act	*Cruzan v. Director* (1990)
Technology Assistance Act	*Troxel v. Granville* (2000)

FAMILY SUPPORT AND FAMILY QUALITY OF LIFE

For the last two decades, the disability field has gradually come to a consensus that providing family support and delivering services using family-centered approaches are important core concepts of disability policy and practice (Turnbull, et al., 2001). It is suggested in the research literature that disability impacts the whole family (Turnbull et al., 2005), that children are served best in the context of their family life (Parish, Pomeranz, Hemp, Rizzola, & Braddock, 2001), and that professionals collaborating with families can better serve the needs of children with disabilities (Dunst, 1997).

It is noted in the family-centered practice literature that the implementation of family-centered services is driven through several important beliefs (Dunst, 2002; Duwa, Wells, & Lalinde, 1993). Chief among these important beliefs are (a) the family rather than the professional is the constant influencing force in the child's life; (b) the family knows best the needs and well-being of the child; (c) the family is the best helper of the child and this help may extend to an understanding of the family's community and to providing information that the family needs; and (d) family participation and decision making in the provision of services, showing respect and affirming families' strengths, enhancing family control over the services they receive, and partnerships and collaborations with families are emphasized (Dempsey & Keen, 2008).

Families who have a member with a disability living at home face extraordinary challenges related to the individual's disability and the family's capacity to provide support. Family support refers to a variety of support, including cash assistance; professionally provided services; in-kind support from other individuals or entities; goods or products; or any combination of services that are provided to families who have minor or adult members with disabilities living in the family's home (Turnbull, Summers, Lee, & Kyzar, 2007). Family support enables families to provide needed support at home and assists them to function as a unit. Family support enhances QOL of families by helping them to be better included in their communities and guiding their member with a disability toward achievement of the nation's goals for people with disabilities. Family support can therefore effectively improve the lives of people with disabilities and their families. Family support policies and practices are more effective when the family and the individual each have the right and opportunity to control the use of funds and determine what and how they are served.

Supporting Families as a Policy Emphasis

Supporting families has become an important public policy for many reasons. First, families are the core units of society and advancing their QOL and ability to have control over their destinies and personal decisions is consistent with long-established constitutional principles of family autonomy and personal liberty. Second, families are essential for securing equality of opportunity for their members with disabilities and launching them toward economic self-sufficiency, independent living, and full participation in society.

Third, whatever benefits a family can also benefit the family member with a disability and vice versa, especially when the individual with a disability lives with his/her family or is dependent upon the care and support of his/her family members on a regular basis. Last, families' needs for support services are increasing as family and community inclusion is encouraged even when the individual has severe and/or multiple disabilities. But the public resources to meet those needs have remained stable or, in some federal or state programs, have decreased (Turnbull et al., 2005). Despite these challenges, family support programs can be effective (see Ainbinder, Blanchard, Singer, Sullivan, Powers, Marquis, et al., 1998; Singer et al., 1999), especially when the family and the individual each have the right and capability to control the respective services they receive and do so in partnership with professionals and federal, state, and local government agencies.

Shift of Emphasis of Family Research

As suggested by Turnbull et al. (2005), one of the important disability policy goals is to support the caregiving efforts of families who have a member with a disability and enhance the QOL of the entire family so that all families will remain the core unit in society. With respect to the knowledge base of this goal, research has been more strongly directed toward describing the caregiving efforts of families and the direct impacts of caregiving on families, rather than enhancing and stabilizing the family as a whole. The bulk of the caregiving research related to individuals with disabilities has focused on elderly parents of individuals with intellectual and developmental disabilities (Essex, Seltzer, & Krauss, 1999; Hayden & Heller, 1997; Heller, Miller, & Factor, 1997; Krauss, Seltzer, Gordon, & Friedman, 1996) and family caregiving of adults with mental illness (Biegel, Sales, & Schulz, 1991; Greenberg, Seltzer, Krauss, & Kim 1997; Lefley, 1996). These studies have typically addressed the outcomes of depression, stress, caregiving burden, and coping. Studies on caregiving have generally tended to find a lack of perceived caregiving burden or psychological distress in elderly parents. Both problem behavior of the individual with intellectual disabilities and the severity of disability appear to be associated with greater caregiving challenges (Essex et al., 1999; Krauss et al., 1996). Interestingly, younger caregivers, as compared to their older counterparts, reported that they had more unmet service needs and experienced significantly more personal burden (Hayden & Heller, 1997).

Over the last 2 decades, many researchers have pointed out a tendency in family research that focuses on negative rather than positive personal and family outcomes (Antonovsky & Sourani, 1988; Helff & Glidden, 1998; McKenzie, 1999; Turnbull et al., 1993). Helff and Glidden (1998) reviewed 60 articles distributed evenly across the three chronological phases of 1971 to 1975, 1983, and 1993 for the extent of negativity and positivity reflected in the research questions and language of the articles. They concluded that there has been a decline in negativity but not concomitant increase in positivity and that most researchers report their family adaptation study results in a predominantly negative tone. However, according to the important policy goal of supporting the caregiving efforts and enhancing the QOL of families, it is necessary to develop a conceptualization and measurement system for the construct of FQoL and to ensure that measures enable positive as well as negative family outcomes to be identified. Leaders in the disability field have called for FQoL as a valued outcome of policies and services (Bailey et al., 1998; Dunst & Bruder, 2002; McKenzie, 1999).

THE DEVELOPMENT OF FAMILY QUALITY OF LIFE

With its roots in the individual QOL concept, FQoL has emerged in response to the needs for a strength-based theoretical and conceptual framework within which to understand and develop family-centered approaches to family support (Brown & Brown, 2004). In 2000, several international research teams met in the World Congress of the International Association for the Scientific Study of Intellectual Disability (IASSID) to share the results of their research endeavors for moving from an individual to a family as the unit of analysis to conceptualize, measure, and apply QOL (Turnbull et al., 2004). Since 1998, researchers at the Beach Center on Disability have initiated a series of qualitative and quantitative studies trying to understand and measure the FQoL construct through the lens of families who have children with disabilities. The results of the series of studies will be reported in detail in the subsequent sections regarding conceptualization and measurement of FQoL. Aside from the Beach Center endeavor, Brown, Anand, Isaacs, Baum, and Fung (2003) from Canada partnered with other international researchers to develop a conceptual framework and a survey instrument for gathering qualitative and quantitative information from families of children with disabilities regarding FQoL. Some of the key work carried out by these international colleagues is summarized below in the sections of conceptualizing and measuring FQoL.

In addition, the IASSID Special Interest Research Group (SIRG) on QOL has contributed to the research development by embracing the topic of FQoL in its annual discussions over the past several years. This group is made up of researchers from a number of countries including Australia, Canada, Holland, Japan, Mexico, the United Kingdom, and the United States. Although the SIRG was initially concerned with the topic of individual QOL, their work on conceptualization, measurement, and application of QOL have greatly influenced the development of FQoL for children with intellectual disabilities. This resulted in the section on "The Family" in a special issue on QOL in the *Journal of Intellectual Disability Research* (Schalock, 2005). Many members of this group worked collaboratively with the researchers at the Beach Center on Disability, and their collaboration led to the first handbook on FQoL published by the American Association on Intellectual and Developmental Disabilities (formerly AAMR; Turnbull et al., 2004). Further work by the QOL-SIRG is to stimulate a wide range of international applied researchers and practitioners who are formulating a wide array of practical recommendations (Brown, Schalock, & Brown, 2009).

Conceptualizing FQoL

FQoL, in a lay sense, involves the goodness of family life. There are many aspects of family life that people everywhere share and in which they strive to attain a satisfactory outcome. Brown and Brown (2004) suggested that numerous important aspects of family life need to be taken into account as people attempted to follow those concepts and principles detailed in individual QOL. They noted that families tend to raise children and mold them into the ways of the family as well as in the broader social and cultural context. Family members want to be healthy and have energy to be active inside and outside the family. Family members like to initiate and accomplish things, both individually and collectively as a whole family. Families like to do things together, for example, to explore and create, to play and laugh, to experience the environment where they live. Families like their members to be closely connected each other, to love, feel compassion, and care for each other. Families also like to interact with other families. Families like to form part of and connect with what their culture has accomplished and carried on its traditions. Families like to transcend everyday experience to dream and to connect with powers that are greater than themselves. Families tend to seek stability in economic, psychological, and social terms even though these attributes may be negated by family and community circumstances.

Despite the fact that families share many characteristics, each family is to some degree unique in terms of its likes and dislikes and things that they consider important. When professionals attempt to understand the concept of FQoL, they need to focus on both aspects of FQoL: the aspect that most families share universally and the aspect that a family values uniquely. In particular, the latter aspect is more important as researchers and practitioners tend to respect the family's voice about what is important to the family.

As mentioned earlier, two research teams have taken separate efforts in developing the FQoL conceptual framework. In a series of studies, researchers at the Beach Center on Disability first conducted a grounded theory qualitative study to explore the perspectives of family members of children and youth with and without disabilities and disability service providers and administrators in defining FQoL (Poston et al., 2003). As a result, these researchers have generated a definition of FQoL delineated as the following: "Families experience a high quality of life when their needs are met, they enjoy their time together, and they are able to do things that are important to them" (Park et al., 2003, p. 367).

The results also revealed a two-facet domain structure: individual-oriented domains and family-oriented domains. The individual-oriented domains represent the idiosyncratic ways of the impact of each individual family member's QOL on the QOL of other family members and on the family as a whole. Similar to many individual QOL domains (Schalock et al., 2002), the six individual-oriented domains of FQoL consist of Advocacy, Emotional Well-being, Health, Physical Environment, Productivity, and Social Well-Being. However, the family-oriented domains represent QOL at the family unit level rather than at the individual family member level, which provide a context within which individual family members interact, reverberate, and live their life collectively as a unit. The four family-oriented domains are Daily Family Life, Family Interaction, Parenting, and Financial Well-being. Nine out of 10 domains are relevant for all families who have children with and without disabilities. The 10th domain, Advocacy, is only relevant for the families who have a member with a disability (Poston et al., 2003). These findings became the basis for developing a measure of FQoL: The Family Quality of Life Scale (FQOLS). Through a series of pilot and national validation studies, the Beach Center researchers have reported an evolution of FQoL domain structure from a 10-domain structure to a 5-domain structure based on factor analysis (Hoffman, Marquis, Poston, Summers, & Turnbull, 2006; Park et al., 2003; Wang, et al., 2004; see a detailed description of the development of FQOLS and evolution of FQoL domain structure in the subsequent section). Summers et al. (2005) concluded that the current Beach Center FQoL conceptual framework consists of five domains: Family Interaction, Parenting, Emotional Well-being, Physical/Material Well-being, and Disability-related Support.

An international research team including researchers mainly from Canada, Australia Israel, and the United States has collaboratively developed another more holistic FQoL conceptual framework based on some of their previous work in individual QOL. These researchers focused the FQoL conceptualization on six aspects or dimensions of life quality across nine major areas of family life (Brown & Brown, 2004; Isaacs et al., 2007). FQoL is defined as the following: "Families experience satisfactory family quality of life when they (a) attain what families everywhere, and they in particular, strive for; (b) are satisfied with what families everywhere, and they in particular, have attained; and (c) feel empowered to live the lives they wish to live" (Brown & Brown, 2004, p. 32). The nine focus areas of family life of children with intellectual disabilities that are modeled after the core domains of individual QOL conceptualization include Health of Family, Financial Well-being, Family Relationships, Support from Other People, Support from Disability-related Services, Spiritual and Cultural Beliefs, Careers and Preparing for Careers, Leisure and Enjoyment of Life, and Community and Civic Involvement. FQoL is represented in all these nine areas from six aspects or dimensions of life quality: Importance, Opportunity, Initiative, Stability, Attainment, and Satisfaction (Isaacs et al., 2007). Importance pertains to the degree to which things or circumstances within any one life area are viewed by families as important. Opportunity refers to the options available to families, for example, opportunities for securing family income or opportunities to take part in leisure activities. Initiative refers to the degree to which families, on their own or with some support, take advantage of available opportunities. Stability refers to the degree to which circumstances within any one life area are likely to improve, decline, or stay the same. Attainment refers to the degree to which the family is able to obtain or accomplish those things that they want or need. Satisfaction is about the overall perception of family members about important aspects of family life.

Measuring FQoL

FQoL, as a multidimensional construct, creates a big challenge for researchers to measure. Although FQoL is the topic of some empirical studies, the measures that were used to measure FQoL have been mostly qualitative in nature (e.g., extensive family interviews; Brown et al., 2003) or have been designed for a specific population (e.g., families of adolescents; Olson & Barnes, 1982). Assessing subjective family well-being via a qualitative method has the advantage of providing a grounded theory-based (Strauss & Corbin, 1990) measure that well reflects the voices of the participants (i.e., families). However, such measures are difficult to use in large-scale theoretical or applied research because qualitative inquiry is very time consuming and requires sophisticated skills to analyze data and interpret the results. In addition, for the sake of assessing FQoL as an overall family outcome measure (Bailey et al., 1998), it is necessary to develop a quantitative instrument that has sound psychometric properties. As a result, two major instruments concerning FQoL were developed separately by different researchers based on different FQoL frameworks. Researchers at the Beach Center on Disability developed the FQOLS through a series of studies funded by the National Institute on Disability and Rehabilitation Research (Park et al., 2003; Poston et al., 2003; Summers et al., 2005). A group of international researchers collaboratively developed the Family Quality of Life Survey (FQoLS; Isaacs et al., 2007).

Family Quality of Life Scale (FQOLS). The FQOLS was developed based on the results of a qualitative study regarding perceptions of families of children and youth with disabilities about FQoL (Poston et al., 2003). Poston et al. pointed out that, as the first phase of a series of studies, the qualitative inquiry was to develop a grounded theory in order to conceptualize and organize the different domains of FQoL. The participating families were asked to describe the factors that help things go well and the factors that contribute to difficult times in their family lives. The themes and subthemes generated through qualitative data analysis were used as the basis for developing 112 items of a pilot scale designed to measure FQoL.

In the second phase of their inquiry series, the researchers at the Beach Center on Disability undertook an initial psychometric evaluation of the pilot version of the FQOLS by using exploratory factor analysis to reduce the items and develop subscales (Park et al., 2003). In the FQOLS, family members were asked to rate the importance and satisfaction of each item related to their overall family life on a 5-point Likert scale. Exploratory factor analysis was used to refine the overall scale and reduce the number of items. To ensure excellent psychometric properties (e.g., convergent validity, internal consistency), Park et al. (2003) removed those items that did not share significant common variance with other items. The exploratory factor analysis resulted in a five-factor solution including four factors referring to the general roles of the family as a social unit (Family Interaction, Parenting, General Resources, Health and Safety) and one concerning family support (Support for Persons with Disabilities). In the third phase of the research program, three studies were conducted to confirm and refine the factor structure and establish further validity and reliability of the scale (Hoffman et al., 2006; Wang et al., 2004, 2006). The Beach Center researchers consistently confirmed a five-factor solution that led to a 25-item scale including five domains of FQoL (two domains renamed): Family Interaction, Parenting, Emotional Well-being, Physical/Material Well-being and Disability Related Support. Item models for each factor had good to excellent model fit for both importance and satisfaction ratings of FQoL (Hoffman et al., 2006). The overall scale structure resulted in excellent fit for the subscale-level models for both importance and satisfaction ratings. Convergent validity measures were significantly correlated with the two subscales of the FQOLS: the Family Adaptability, Partnership, Growth, Affection, and Resolve (APGAR) (Smilkstein, Ashworth, & Montano, 1982) to the Family Interaction subscale and Family Resource Scale (Dunst & Leet, 1985) to the Physical/Material Well-being subscale. Test–retest reliability correlations were significant for both importance and satisfaction ratings for all subscales of the FQOLS (Hoffman et al., 2006). Therefore, Hoffman et al. concluded that the FQOLS is a valid, authentic and efficient device for assessing the impact of services on families. Such scales have the potential to serve as an outcome measure at many different levels and may be useful to various stakeholders in research, policy, and service sectors who are working to make substantial and sustainable enhancements in the QOL of families who have children with disabilities.

Family Quality of Life Survey (FQoLS). The development of another instrument, the FQoLS based in Canada, has involved colleagues from a number of countries including Australia, Israel, and the United States. As described earlier, the FQoLS collects both qualitative and quantitative data on nine areas of family life, including Health of the Family, Financial Well-being, Family Relationships, Support from Other People, Support from Disability-related Services, Spiritual and Cultural Beliefs, Careers and Preparing for Careers, Leisure and Enjoyment of life, and Community and Civic Involvement. Within each of these nine areas or domains, questions are asked in terms of six dimensions, Importance, Opportunity, Initiative, Attainment, Stability, and Satisfaction (Isaacs et al., 2007). Two out of six dimensions are specific outcome measures, Family Attainment and Family Satisfaction. They measure family perceived attainment and satisfaction in all the nine areas/domains of family life. The additional explanatory measures are Importance, Opportunities, Initiative, and Stability. Early work in developing the FQoLS suggested that these dimensions largely encapsulated the interests and concerns of families and are, therefore, germane to an understanding of practical needs and support in the specific areas outlined above. It is also noted that the FQoLS has a life span orientation and appears culturally sensitive as it is being applied in an increasing number of countries. The validation studies of the FQoLS psychometric properties are under way, with data collection efforts in a number of countries, and preliminary findings regarding the reliability and validity of FQoLS have been reported (Wang, Samuel, Isaacs, Baum, & Brown, 2008).

Application of FQoL

The concept of FQoL can be applied constructively in a number of contexts. Brown and Brown (2004) suggested that FQoL should become an ultimate goal of work aimed at assisting and supporting families in need. FQoL represents a new perspective for organizing positive value concerning families and has become a guiding principle for policy development, service delivery, and family support and interventions in the field of disability. With the embracement of the FQoL concept, researchers and practitioners have begun to adopt a new vision for studying and supporting families through partnership with families (Turnbull & Turnbull, 2003).

Social service agencies and family support organizations can use each of the FQoL measures at the family level for family need assessment and at the program level for assessment of service effectiveness and program evaluation. In terms of family level usage, both FQOLS and FQoLS are family-friendly surveys that can be used collaboratively with families in planning for delivery of family-centered services and supports. In particular, such tools might be completed by families in a rating checklist format. The FQoL domains and indicators could be used as probes in interviews or conversations with families in gathering open-ended information. For example, the Beach Center Family Quality of Life Conversation Guide, available for free at the Beach Center's Web site (http://www.beachcenter.org/resource_library/), is a useful tool to assist families and professionals (e.g., service coordinators, case managers, or others) to think through the family's needs for support and services. The FQoLS also has many specific qualitative survey questions for gathering important family information. It is available for free of charge (http://www.surreyplace.on.ca/Content/File/FQOL Survey General Version Without Variable Names May 08.pdf). Both FQOLS and FQoLS can provide families and professionals a step-by-step process to consider the needs of a family in each of the domains and items within domains. Families can then be guided to consider whether a need has a low, medium, or high priority in terms of getting help and support to meet their needs. Agency administrators who seek to enhance their program effectiveness in improving family outcomes can benefit from having aggregated data across all families being served concerning families' ratings of importance and satisfaction of various FQoL domains and indicators.

However, there are caveats about quantifying the evaluation solely based on the FQoL survey scores. Authors of both FQOLS and FQoLS have argued against using a single total FQoL score for clinical purposes because of families' concerns. Families do not want to be perceived as having a "FQoL quotient" that would deem them as "dysfunctional" if they receive a low score in FQOLS. They do not want loss of supports and services if they score too high in FQOLS. Indeed, a single FQoL score would not help to identify specific strengths and weaknesses in family lives (Poston et al.,

2003). It is the use of domain specifics (e.g., qualitative commentary of individual respondents that identify the specific aspects of domain rating) and dimension analysis that helps to identify areas of need (Brown, 2006a).

Summers et al. (2005) suggested that the short-term outcomes of supports and services (e.g. empowerment) lead to the ultimate outcome of FQoL. Therefore, agencies may want to use specifically tailored measures to assess these short-term outcomes and be held accountable only for the supports and services they provide, while simultaneously assessing the overall, long-term outcome, FQoL, with a common FQoL measure. This approach to identifying and assessing outcomes could have policy and practice advantages in that it would allow for comparisons across types of supports, services, and settings. This is an area where further research should be directed.

For the same purpose of assessing the family's needs in correspondence with support and services, FQoLS has been used both as a measure for identifying needs of families and as an outcome measure of family support and services (Isaacs et al., 2007). For example, based on the data from Australia, Canada, Taiwan, and South Korea collected through an earlier version of FQoLS, Brown (2006) noted that a number of similar trends emerged, though at different levels, in terms of satisfaction across the nine domains of FQoL. In the Korean data of families with children with intellectual disabilities ($n=73$, mean age $=7.7$ years, and $SD=2.3$), families' satisfaction with FQoL rose above 50% only in one domain, Family Relations (Hong, 2005). In the data from Taiwan of families of children with autism ($n=83$, mean age of children $=5.4$ years), no single FQoL domain recorded 50% satisfaction (Wang, 2003). In the Canadian data of families of children with intellectual disabilities ($n=51$, mean age $=7.7$ years), families' ratings on FQoL rose above 50% satisfaction only for the domains of Health, Family Relations, and Spiritual and Cultural Beliefs (Brown, MacAdam-Crisp, Wang, & Iaroci, 2006). In the Australian sample (reported by Brown, 2006b), which represents a mixed intellectual disability group ($n=55$), families reported over the 50% satisfaction level on five FQoL domains including Health, Family Relations, Spiritual and Cultural Beliefs, Careers and Preparing for Careers, and Leisure and Enjoyment of Life. However, the overall pattern of satisfaction scores (i.e., highs and lows) were very similar for the two groups. Some data from older parents in Canada also showed higher satisfaction levels (Jokinen & Brown, 2005). Families' satisfaction with disability services in each country was the lowest or among the lowest of the FQoL domain scores. This trend suggests that families, regardless of country of origin, are dissatisfied with the disability service due to either the lack of disability service or the quality of service they received.

Although an enormous amount of work remains to be carried out on country and cultural issues in relation to FQoL, it does appear that some common trends and differences are beginning to emerge. Wang et al.

(2004) suggested that the level of satisfaction may be related to the form (type and severity) of disability, particularly when a child has major behavioral challenges. Despite considerable variation of the level of satisfaction with the FQoL domains across cultures and countries, financial issues for the family, careers and orientation for careers, and support from disability-related service seem to be common vulnerable areas of family life regardless of geographic origin. The message for professionals is clear that the commonly rated low satisfaction areas by families are critical to consider as the priority of improvement in services and supports. Attention should also be paid to the qualitative data of each family collected via FQoLS. Practitioners and researchers can ascertain the critical issues that precipitate low satisfaction in single-family cases by exploring the qualitative data from different family respondents.

IMPLICATIONS FOR THE FIELD OF SOCIAL WORK

Researchers can learn what policy makers, program administrators, and service providers can do to make a difference in the lives of families of individuals with disabilities. One valuable social work function would be to look for attributes, needs, and processes that have the greatest positive impact on FQoL and then provide resources to families and professionals to make things happen to stabilize and improve FQoL.

Families are the core units of society and have extraordinary caregiving responsibilities for their members with disabilities. Although families sometimes prefer to keep their families intact and avoid out-of-home care, federal and state policy and practice should respond to perceived family needs by providing funds and services to families. Research has demonstrated that families who have members with intellectual disabilities living in the family home have broader family needs as a result of having a member with a disability. The number of such families may well be changing, yet the amount and intensity of support for the families of individuals with disabilities as a whole is not.

The field of social work, like many other disciplines or professions, has embraced the rhetoric of family-centered services and the enhancement of family outcomes for decades. However, the important next step for the field of social work is to match the rhetoric with a conceptual framework that can guide the evolution of research and family support over time to ultimately produce significant and sustainable enhancements in families' outcomes. The FQoL construct can provide an overarching framework for conceptualizing social problems, planning intervention strategies, guiding practices, and evaluating outcomes of programs. As research and practice become more closely conjoined through evidence-based models, the conceptual framework of FQoL has great potential to be an organizing force for the theoretical bases and practice principles informing social work interventions.

Brown and Brown (2003) have provided detailed practical recommendations based on QOL studies. Any QOL model, if it is to empower families, has to take into account the issue of personal values. In this case it is the family's values. Social work professionals need to carefully evaluate their proposed actions in terms of the family value system and ensure their own personal value system does not distort proposed actions. Many examples were provided in Brown and Brown (2003) that revealed professional, family, and individual dilemmas posed by ethical and professional challenges in a world where variability, choice, self-image, and self-actualization are important.

Choices made by any family may be based on a wide range of issues arising from family dynamics. The role of the professional is to help families dissect their motivations and help a family recognize how the person with a disability may influence their individual and family choices. For example, it is noted that in families where a child with a disability is present, the mother, in particular, frequently directs attention to that child, sometimes at the expense of other family members (Brown et al., 2006). The choices made by mothers or other members of the family may be viable and appropriate, but they will often need to be renegotiated based on the internal constructs and needs of the family. The professional's role is to help the family examine these, with the aim of increasing motivation and helping family members to take control and make decisions that enhance and reinforce family and individual values. The application of FQoL should enhance the degree of family control and opportunities with respect to their activities and environments. This may mean frequently changing service options or redesigning new options for support for the family as well as the individual with a disability. For example, a family may choose to heighten its economic power through the mother working for pay. Support may mean providing resources for her to do this, so the needs of the child with a disability can be met and, at the same time, the mother can increase her skills and knowledge, heightening her self-image and the economic resources of the family. It is important to recognize that such decisions often have long-term impacts, and therefore one is assisting the family invest in their distant future as well as present circumstances. The above underscores several features of the FQoL framework: choice, fulfillment, and empowerment. Professionals such as social workers, albeit honoring the family's values, should not avoid their responsibility to influence or intervene when the family shows that they have a negative attitude to or make inappropriate decisions for the family member with a disability. The FQoL framework sees it as important for professionals to help the family members to reflect their own value systems and understand other value systems. Brown et al. (1992) found in a longitudinal study that families who believed their children could improve did so to a greater extent than families who did not think their children would improve; they also found that family members whose children received support based on a QOL framework did better than similar parents who did not receive such supports. Not only does this argue for a FQoL approach, but it also underscores the importance of helping family members to reflect their value systems and willingly change their attitude toward a positive outlook when the family does not have one.

Recommendations

A number of recommendations flow from this work. First, social workers and allied professionals need to consider using a FQoL survey or scale to gain information about a family's overall satisfaction with their family life across domains. Within this assessment structure, they need to look for specific commentary. In several of the studies quoted above, family members commented, for example, "We can not obtain respite when required; my husband and I have not been out together for the past 15 years, nor have any of us had a vacation since our child with autism was born"; "I gave up a lucrative career to spend more time at home to support my wife"; "I was studying for social work when I gave birth to my child with autism. I have now had to give up studying because I do not know how to cope."

Second, social workers and allied professionals should look for strengths and weakness in family domains among family members. Third, social workers should be aware that some families record satisfaction when they still need support. For example, it appears that older parents may record higher satisfaction levels than younger parents, but may have increasing health support needs (Jokinen & Brown, 2005). Fourth, social workers should consider likely future domain needs for the family. Anticipation and organization can reduce the development of extreme situations. Fifth, social workers should look for ways of supporting the family, not just the child with a disability. For example, they can help look for funds for a career mother who wants to study, look for respite care so that the parents can go out together from time to time, and discuss with the family about types of relief required to ensure other siblings can grow and develop positively. Sixth, social workers should recognize that there are large differences in satisfaction across FQoL domains. Some families have an overall satisfaction with their family life because of having a child with a disability in the family, particularly where gross behavioral disturbance does not occur.

Last, although the idea of taking families into account when planning service delivery and giving families a real role in the process of evaluating service quality is not new to the field of social work, much hard work, advocacy, and challenge still lie ahead. There is a perceived need to change policies in response to those challenges. Social workers should not only assist the service delivery system in changing their structure but also advocate in alliance with families for policy change toward the enhancement of FQoL for families of children with disabilities. Researchers in the field should pay attention to studying how specific policy directives and practices at the local agency level are shaped and influenced by state and federal policies that embrace the FQoL concept and principles to address the service needs of families of individuals with disabilities.

REFERENCES

Ainbinder, J., Blanchard, L., Singer, G. H. S., Sullivan, M., Powers, L., Marquis, J., & Santelli, B. (1998). How parents help one another: A qualitative study of parent to parent self-help. *Journal of Pediatric Psychology, 23*, 99–109.

Andrews, A. B., & Ben-Arieh, A. (1999). Measuring and monitoring children's well-being across the world. *Social Work, 44*(2), 105–114.

Antonovsky, A., & Sourani, T. (1988). Family sense of coherence and family adaptation. *Journal of Marriage and the Family, 50*, 79–82.

Arad, B. D. (2001). Parental features and quality of life in the decision to remove children at risk from home. *Child Abuse & Neglect, 25*, 47–64.

Bailey, D. B., McWilliam, R. A., Darkes, L. A., Hebbeler, K., Simeonsson, R. J., Spiker, D., & Wagner. (1998). Family outcomes in early intervention: A framework for program evaluation and efficacy research. *Exceptional Children, 64*, 313–328.

Biegel, D. E., Sales, E., & Schulz, R. (1991). Family caregiving in chronic illness: Alzheimer's disease, cancer, heart disease, mental illness, and stroke (Vol. 1). In D. Biegel & R. Schulz (Eds.), *Family Caregiver Applications Series*. Newbury Park, CA: Sage.

Blake, W. M., & Anderson, D. C. (2000). Quality of life: Perceptions of African Americans. *Journal of Black Studies, 30*(3), 411–427.

Brown, R. I. (Ed.). (1997). *Quality of life for people with disabilities* (2nd ed.). Cheltenham, UK: Stanley Thornes.

Brown, R. I. (2006a). Editorial. *Journal of Policy and Practice in Intellectual Disabilities, 3*(4), 209–210.

Brown, R. I. (2006a, August). International research in Family quality of life. Paper presented at the IASSID European Conference, Mastricht, Holland.

Brown, I., Anand, S., Isaacs, B., Baum, N., & Fung, W. L. (2003). Family quality of life: Canadian results from an international study. *Journal of Developmental and Physical Disabilities, 15*(3), 207–230.

Brown, R. I., Bayer, M. B., & MacFarlane, C. (1989). *Rehabilitation programs: Performance and quality of life of adults with developmental handicaps*. Toronto, Canada: Lugus.

Brown, R. I., Bayer, M. B., & Brown, P. M. (1992). *Empowerment and developmental handicaps: Choices and quality of life*. Toronto, Canada: Captus.

Brown, I., & Brown, R. (2003). *Quality of life and disability: An approach for community practitioners*. London: Jessica Kingsley.

Brown, I., & Brown, R. (2004). Family quality of life as an area of study. In A. Turnbull, I. Brown & R. Turnbull (Eds.), *Families and persons with mental retardation and quality of life: International perspectives*. Washington, DC: American Association on Mental Retardation.

Brown, R. I., MacAdam-Crisp, J., Wang, M., & Iaroci, G. (2006). Family quality of life when there is a child with a developmental disability. *Journal of Policy and Practice in Intellectual Disabilities, 3*(4), 238–245.

Brown, R. I., Schalock, R. L., & Brown, I. (2009). Concept of quality of life and its application to persons with intellectual disabilities and their families: Introduction and overview. *Journal of Policy and Practice in Intellectual Disabilities, 6*(1), 1–5.

Carter, E. A., & McGoldrick, M. (Eds.). (1989). *The changing family life cycle: A framework for family therapy* (2nd ed.). Boston: Allyn & Bacon.

Chipuer, H. M., Bramston, P., & Pretty, G. (2003). Determinants of subjective quality of life among rural adolescents: A developmental perspective. *Social Indicators Research, 61*, 79–95.

Cummins, R. A. (1997a). Assessing quality of life. In R. I. Brown (Ed.), *Quality of life for people with disabilities: Models, research and practice* (pp. 116–150). Cheltenham, UK: Stanley Thornes.

Cummins, R. A.. (1997b). *Comprehensive Quality of Life Scale Intellectual/Cognitive Disability.* School of Psychology, Deakin University, Australia.

Deardorff, K., & Hollman, F. (1997). *U.S. population estimates by age, sex, race, and Hispanic origin: 1990 to 1996.* Washington, DC: U.S. Government Printing Office.

Dempsey, I., & Keen, D. (2008). A review of processes and outcomes in family-centered services for children with a disability. *Topics in Early Childhood Special Education, 28*(1), 42–52.

Dunst, C. J. (1997). Conceptual and empirical foundations of familycentered practice. In R. J. Illback, C. T. Cobb, & H. M. Joseph, Jr. (Eds.), *Integrated services for children and families: Opportunities for psychological practice* (pp. 75–91). Washington, DC: American Psychological Association.

Dunst, C. J. (2002). Family-centered practices: Birth through high school. *Journal of Special Education, 36*, 139–147.

Dunst, C. J., & Bruder, M. B. (2002). Valued outcomes of service coordination, early intervention, and natural environments. *Exceptional Children, 68*(3), 361–375.

Dunst, C. J., & Leet, H. E. (1985). *Family resource scale: Reliability and validity.* Asheville, NC: Winterberry Press.

Duwa, S. M., Wells, C., & Lalinde, P. (1993). Creating family-centered programs and policies. In D. M. Bryant & M. A. Graham (Eds.), *Implementing early intervention: From research to effective practice* (pp. 99–123). New York: Guilford.

Essex, E. L., Seltzer, M. M., & Krauss, M. W. (1999). Differences in coping effectiveness and well-being among aging mothers and fathers of adults with retardation. *American Journal of Mental Retardation, 104*(6), 545–563.

Evandrou, M., & Glaser, K. (2004). Family, work and quality of life: Changing economic and social roles through the life course. *Ageing and Society, 24*(5), 771–791.

Felce, D. (1997). Defining and applying the concept of quality of life. *Journal of Intellectual Disability Research, 41*(2), 126–135.

Fujiura, G. T., & Yamaki, K. (2000). Trends in demography of childhood poverty and disability. *Exceptional Children, 66*, 187–199.

Gettys, G. D. (1980). *Black families' residential choice and quality of life.* PhD dissertation, Bryn Mawr College, Graduate School of Social Work and Social

Research. Retrieved June 15, 2008, from Dissertations & Theses: Full Text database. (Publication No. AAT 8103907).

Gitlin, L. N., Reever, K., Dennis, M. P., Mathieu, E., & Hauck, W. W. (2006). Enhancing quality of life of families who use adult day services: Short- and long-term effects of the adult day services plus program. *The Gerontologist*, *46*(5), 630–639.

Goode, D. A. (Ed.). (1994). *Quality of life for persons with disabilities: International perspectives and issues*. Cambridge, MA: Brookline.

Greenberg, J., Seltzer, M. M., Krauss, M. W., & Kim, H. W. (1997). The differential effects of social support on the psychological well-being of aging mothers of adults with mental illness or mental retardation. *Family Relations*, *46*, 383–394.

Hansson, L. (2002). Quality of life in depression and anxiety. *International Review of Psychiatry*, *14*, 185–189.

Hayden, M. F., & Heller, T. (1997). Support, problem-solving/coping ability, and personal burden of younger and older caregivers of adults with mental retardation. *Mental Retardation*, *35*, 364–372.

Helff, C. M., & Glidden, L. M. (1998). More positive or less negative? Trends in research on adjustment of families rearing children with developmental disabilities. *Mental Retardation*, *36*(6), 457–464.

Heller, T., Miller, A. B., & Factor, A. (1997). Adults with mental retardation as supports to their parents: Effects on parental caregiving appraisal. *Mental Retardation*, *35*, 338–346.

Hoffman, L., Marquis, J. G., Poston, D. J., Summers, J. A., & Turnbull, A. P. (2006). Assessing family outcomes: Psychometric evaluation of the family quality of life scale. *Journal of Marriage and Family*, *68*, 1069–1083.

Holloway, F., & Carson, J. (2002). Quality of life in severe mental illness. *International Review of Psychiatry*, *14*, 175–184.

Hong, K. (2005). *Family quality of life in South Korea*. Paper presented at Quality of Life Special Interest Group of International Association for the Scientific Study of Intellectual Disabilities, Round Table Meeting: Vancouver, Canada.

Hughes, C., & Hwang, B.. (1996). Attempts to conceptualize and measure quality of life. In R. L. Schalock (Ed.), *Quality of life, vol. 1: Conceptualization and measurement* (pp. 51–61). Washington, DC: American Association on Mental Retardation.

Ihinger-Tallman, M. (1995). Quality of life and well-being of single parent families: Disparate voices or a long overdue chorus? *Marriage and Family Review*, *20*(3/4), 513–532.

Isaacs, B. J., Brown, I., Brown, R. I., Baum, N., Myerscough, T., Neikrug, S., et al. (2007). The international family quality of life project: Goals and description of a survey tool. *Journal of Policy and Practice in Intellectual Disabilities*, *4*(3), 177–185.

Jokinen, N. S., & Brown, R. I. (2005). Family quality of life from the perspective of older parents. *Journal of Intellectual Disability Research*, *49*(10), 789–793.

Krauss, M. W., Seltzer, M. M., Gordon, R., & Friedman, D. H. (1996). Binding ties: The roles of adult siblings of persons with mental retardation. *Mental Retardation*, *34*(2), 83–93.

Kutner, N. G., Mistretta, E. F., & Barnhart, H. X. (1999). Family members' perceptions of quality of life change in dementia SCU residents. *Journal of Applied Gerontology*, *18*(4), 423–439.

Lefley, H. (1996). Family caregiving for adults with mental illness (Vol. 7). In D. Biegel & R. Schulz (Eds.), *Family caregiver applications series*. Newbury Park, CA: Sage.

Lowenstein, A.. (2007). Solidarity-conflict and ambivalence: Testing two conceptual frameworks and their impact on quality of life for older family members. *Journals of Gerontology*, Series B: Psychological Sciences and Social Sciences, *62B*(2), S100–S107.

Mactavish, J. B., MacKay, K. J., & Iwasaki, Y. (2007). Family caregivers of individuals with intellectual disability: Perspectives on life quality and the role of vacations. *Journal of Leisure Research*, *39*(1), 127–155.

McKenzie, S. (1999). Using quality of life as the focus for investigating the lives of people who have children with disabilities. *International Journal of Practical Approaches to Disability*, *23*(2), 9–16.

Meuleners, L. B., Lee, A. H., Binns, C. W., & Lower, A. (2003). Quality of life for adolescents: Assessing measurement properties using structural equation modeling. *Quality of Life Research*, *12*, 283–290.

Nandi, P. K., & Harris, H. (1999). The social world of female-headed families: A study of quality of life in a marginalized neighborhood. *International Journal of Comparative Sociology*, *40*(2), 195–214.

National Association of Social Workers. (NASW). (2002). *NASW standards for school social work services*. Washington, DC: Author.

NASW. (2003). *NASW standards for the practice of social work with adolescents*. Washington, DC: Author.

NASW. (2005). *NASW standards for social work practice in child welfare*. Washington, DC: Author.

National Research Council. (2002). *Minority students in special and gifted education*. Washington, DC: National Academy Press.

Olson, D. H., & Barnes, H. L. (1982). Quality of life. In D. H. Olson, H. I. McCubbin, H. Barnes, A. Larsen, M. Muxen, & M. Wilson (Eds.), *Family inventories* (pp. 55–67). Minneapolis, MN: Life Innovations.

Parish, S. L., Pomeranz, A., Hemp, R., Rizzola, M. C., & Braddock, D. (2001). *Family support for persons with developmental disabilities in the U.S.: Status and trends* (Policy Research Brief). Minneapolis: University of Minnesota, Institute on Community Integration.

Park, J., Marquis, J., Hoffman, L., Turnbull, A., Poston, D., Mannan, H., et al. (2003). Assessing the family quality of life as the service outcome. *Journal of Intellectual Disability Research*, *47*(5), 367–384.

Poston, D., Turnbull, A., Park, J., Mannan, H., Marquis, J., & Wang, M. (2003). Family quality of life: A qualitative inquiry. *Mental Retardation*, *41*(5), 313–328.

Raphael, D., Renwick, R., & Brown, I. (1997). *Quality of Life Instrument Package for adults with developmental disabilities*. Quality of Life Research Unit, Centre for Health Promotion, University of Toronto.

Renwick, R., Brown, I., & Nagler, M. (1996). *Quality of life in health promotion and rehabilitation: Conceptual approaches, issues, and applications*. Thousand Oaks, CA: Sage.

Rodgers, R. H., & White, J. M. (1993). Family development theory. In P. J. Boss, W. J. Doherty, R. LaRossa, W. R. Schumm & S. K. Steinmetz (Eds.), *Sources of family theories and methods: A contextual approach* (pp. 225–254). New York: Plenum.

Sar, B. K. (1994). *The relationship between task performance and perceived quality of life of families with adopted special-needs children.* PhD dissertation, Virginia Commonwealth University. Retrieved June 15, 2008, from Dissertations & Theses: Full Text database. (Publication No. AAT 9507150)

Schalock, R. L. (2000). Three decades of quality of life. In M. Wehmeyer & J. R. Patton (Eds.), *Mental retardation in the 21st century* (pp. 335–356). Austin, TX: PRO-ED.

Schalock, R. L. (2005). Introduction and overview. Guest editorial. Quality of life [Special issue]. *Journal of Intellectual Disability Research*, *49*(10), 695–698.

Schalock, R. L., Brown, I., Brown, R. I., Cummins, R. A., Felce, D., Matikka, L., et al. (2002). Conceptualization, measurement, and application of quality of life for persons with intellectual disabilities: Report of an international panel of experts. *Mental Retardation*, *40*, 457–470.

Schalock, R. L., & Keith, K. D. (1993). *Quality of life questionnaire*. Worthington, OH: IDS.

Schalock, R. L., & Verdugo, M. A. (2002). *Handbook on quality of life for human service practitioners*. Washington, DC: American Association on Mental Retardation.

Singer, G. H. S., Marquis, J., Powers, L., Blanchard, L., DiVenere, N., Santelli, B., & Sharp, M. (1999). A multi-site evaluation of parent to parent programs for parents of children with disabilities. *Journal of Early Intervention*, *22*(3), 217–229.

Smilkstein, G., Ashworth, C., & Montano, D. (1982). Validity and reliability of the Family APGAR as a test of family function. *Journal of Family Practice*, *15*, 303–311.

Strauss, A., & Corbin, J. (1990). *Basics of qualitative research: Grounded theory procedures and techniques*. Newbury Park, CA: Sage.

Summers, J. A., Poston, D. J., Turnbull, A. P., Marquis, J., Hoffman, L., Mannan, H., et al. (2005). Conceptualizing and measuring family quality of life. *Journal of International Disability Research*, *49*, 777–783.

Teno, J. M., Mor, V., & Ward, N. (2005). Bereaved family member perceptions of quality of end-of-life care in U.S. regions with high and low usage of intensive care unit care. *Journal of the American Geriatrics Society*, *53*(11), 1905–1911.

Troxel v. Granville, 530 U.S. 57 (2000).

Turnbull, H. R., Beegle, G., & Stowe, M. S. (2001). The core concepts of disability policy affecting families who have children with disabilities. *Journal of Disability Policy Studies*, *12*(3), 133–143.

Turnbull, A. P., Brown, I., & Turnbull, R. H., III (Eds.). (2004). *Families and persons with mental retardation and quality of life: International perspectives*. Washington, DC: American Association on Mental Retardation.

Turnbull, A. P., Patterson, J. M., Behr, S. K., Marphy, D. L., Marquis, J. G., & Blue-Banning, M. J. (Eds.). (1993). *Cognitive coping, families, and disability: Participatory action research in action*. Baltimore, MD: Paul H. Brookes.

Turnbull, A. P., & Turnbull, H. R. (2001a). *Families, professionals, and exceptionality: Collaborating for empowerment* (4th ed.). Upper Saddle River, NJ: Merrill/Prentice Hall.

Turnbull, A., & Turnbull, R. (2001b). Self-determination for individuals with significant cognitive disabilities and their families. *Journal of the Association for Persons with Severe Handicaps*, *26*(1), 56–62.

Turnbull, A. P., & Turnbull, H. R. (2003). From the old to the new paradigm of disability and families: Research to enhance family quality of life outcomes. In J. L. Paul, C. D. Lavely, A. Cranston-Gingras & E. L. Taylor (Eds.), *Rethinking professional issues in special education* (pp. 83–117). Westport, CT: Ablex.

Turnbull, A., Turnbull, H. R., Agosta, J., Erwin, E., Fujiura, G., Singer, G., & Soodak, L. (2005). Support of families and family life across the lifespan. In C. Lakin & A. P. Turnbull (Eds.), *National goals and research for persons with intellectual and developmental disabilities* (pp. 217–256). Washington, DC: AAMR.

Turnbull, A. P., Summers, J. A., Lee, S., & Kyzar, K. (2007). Conceptualization and measurement of family outcomes associated with families of individuals with intellectual disabilities. *Mental Retardation and Developmental Disabilities Research Reviews*, *13*(4), 346–356.

Verdugo, M. A., & Schalock R. L. (2003). *Cross-cultural survey of quality of life indicators*. Salamanca, Spain: Institute on Community Integration, Faculty of Psychology.

Wang, M., Samuel, P., Isaacs, B. J., Baum, N., & Brown, I. (2008). *Examining the factor structure of FQoL Survey*. Paper presented at the IASSID Congress, Cape Town, South Africa.

Wang, M., Summers, J. A., Little, T., Turnbull, A., Poston, D., & Mannan, H. (2006). Perspectives of fathers and mothers of children in early intervention programs in assessing family quality of life. *Journal of Intellectual Disability Research*, *50*, 977–988.

Wang, M., Turnbull, A. P., Summers, J. A., Little, T. D., Poston, D. J., Mannan, H., et al. (2004). Severity of disability and income as predictors of parents' satisfaction with their family quality of life during early childhood years. *Research & Practice for Persons with Severe Disabilities*, *29*, 82–94.

Wang, S.-Y. (2003). Family quality of life where there is a child with Autism in Taiwan. Personal correspondence.

World Health Organization Quality of Life Assessment (WHOQOL) Group. (1998). The World Health Organization Quality of Life Assessment (WHOQOL): Development and general psychometric properties. *Social Science and Medicine*, *46*, 1569–1585.

Whitechurch, G. G., & Constantine, L. L. (1993). Systems theory. In P. J. Boss, W. J. Doherty, R. LaRossa, W. R. Schumm & S. K. Steinmetz (Eds.), *Sourcebook of family theories and methods: A contextual approach* (pp. 325–352). New York: Plenum Press.

Wisconsin v. Yoder, 406 U.S. 205 (1972).

Trends Impacting Public Policy Support for Caregiving Families

GEORGE H. S. SINGER
Gevirtz Graduate School of Education, University of California, Santa Barbara, California

DAVID E. BIEGEL
Mandel School of Applied Social Sciences, Case Western Reserve University, Cleveland, Ohio

BRANDY L. ETHRIDGE
Gevirtz Graduate School of Education, University of California, Santa Barbara, California

Public policy aimed at supporting the caregiving capacity of families has risen to prominence on the public agenda in the United States. Initiatives at the state and federal levels have created some initial services. Three trends that are pushing the issue of family caregiving to the surface are discussed, including large-scale social, demographic, and economic changes. The pressures on women from increased caregiving demands are discussed, along with the taken-for-granted cultural value placed on the home as a locus of care for family members who need assistance with common daily activities. Experiments at the state level with consumer-directed care and capitated wrap-around services are described. The authors argue that support for caregiving families is likely to remain a prominent concern of the public and policy makers for the foreseeable future.

Support for caregiving families has gradually risen to prominence on the pubic agenda because of large-scale and persistent societal trends and forces. The purpose of this article is to discuss these trends and forces and their implications for public support for caregiving families. Three major topics are addressed: (1) demographic and economic pressures that bring this issue to the forefront, (2) values influencing public initiatives and design of services, and (3) recent convergence on similar solutions to supporting families regardless of the disabilities or ages of family members needing long-term care.

SOCIAL, DEMOGRAPHIC, AND ECONOMIC STRESSORS

Families in the United States play a pervasive and essential role caregiving for family members with disabilities (Biegel, Sales, & Schulz, 1991). Roughly 30% of the adult U.S. population provides care to a relative or friend who is either frail and/or elderly, and/or has a physical, mental, or emotional disability. Families provide care for children with chronic physical illness and individuals with developmental disabilities, for family members with serious mental illness, and for elderly who require assistance to live independently (National Alliance for Caregiving [NAC], 2009). Most recipients of care had sustained needs, so the average duration of caregiving was 4.6 years, with 31% of caregivers providing care for five or more years (NAC, 2009). Many family caregivers affirmatively choose their role as opposed to simply lacking alternatives. Recent research on parenting children with developmental disabilities and studies of caregiving for elderly family members reveals that, under the right conditions, the givers and receivers of informal family care find benefits (Hastings & Taunt, 2002). As discussed in this article, however, the right conditions for promoting positive outcomes for family caregivers and receivers are often not in place. Under difficult circumstances, caregiving can exact substantial financial, physical, psychological, and social costs (Hughes, Gobbie-Hurder, Weaver, & Hendersen, 1999). In the NAC (2009) survey of a representative sample of caregivers, 31% described themselves as highly stressed, 17% with fair or poor health, and 70% reported that their caregiving responsibilities led to role strain as workers that included such things as reduced work hours or taking a leave of absence. Recent meta-analyses of large numbers of studies found negative impacts on caregivers' health and well-being (Pinquart & Sörensen, 2004; Schulze & Rössler, 2005; Singer, 2006). However, the finding that roughly one third of caregivers experienced uplifts from caregiving suggests that policy makers can aim to not only alleviate stress in caregivers but also to more affirmatively create conditions so that all caregivers can realize the benefits of caregiving for themselves as well as for their care recipients.

The more help that a care recipient requires in basic activities of daily living, the higher the level of caregiver stress (MetLife Mature Market Institute [MMI], 2006; NAC, 2009). Caregivers who are most likely to be injured or experience stress-related problems such as depression are primarily the one third of caregivers who report a high burden of care. Burden, as measured in the NAC study (2009), used an index that included the number of activities for which a care recipient needs help, the number of hours of caregiving per week, and the physical difficulty of providing caregiving. Caregivers who are at highest risk help a loved one with two or more major activities of daily living (e.g., transfer into or out of bed, bathe, dress, or eat) and provide 20 hours or more of caregiving a week. A national advocacy movement has arisen as people seek a collective way to make caregiving less of a burden and more of a natural part of family life. Over the next two decades, as the percentage of elderly citizens and individuals of all ages with disabilities increases, family caregiving and its role in long-term care of people with disabilities is likely to rise in prominence on the national political agenda.

Discussions of public policy for long-term care take place against a backdrop of cultural and historical values entailing assumptions largely taken for granted until called into question by changing realities. We discuss three major historical and cultural background variables affecting family caregiving policy: (1) residualism, (2) a gender bias for allocation of unpaid or underpaid caregiving work to women, and (3) the concept *home* as the preferred place for living a life marked by self-determination and individualism.

RESIDUALISM

Unlike most other countries with advanced economies and high per capita incomes, the United States has been reluctant to build a welfare state and has usually done so in small incremental steps punctuated by large-scale policy changes at rare moments in history. The approach to social welfare, including public allocation of resources to assist family caregivers, has been based on an implicit philosophy of *residualism* (Orloff, 2002). In this value system, it is expected that people must take care of themselves and their families in the event of misfortune. The taken-for-granted assumption inherited from the English Poor Laws is that public resources are provided only after the private social safety net has failed and then only for a small residual number of individuals who require rescue from dire circumstances. For example, elderly individuals and younger people with some disabilities are eligible for Supplemental Security Income (SSI) through the Social Security system, but only if they have liquid assets worth less than US $2,000 for an individual or $3,000 if married (Social Security Administration, 2010). In addition to requisite impoverishment, residualism has also resulted in a bias toward paying for the costs of congregate care institutions instead of home living in the community, even though the vast majority of people with disabilities live in family homes.

Women as Caregivers and the Value of Home as the Locus for Care

Dramatic social and demographic changes over the past century have affected the way work was previously allocated in family homes. These trends include smaller families, increases in the percentage of single-parent families, more childless couples and unmarried adults, and the impoverishment of many women associated with single parenthood and the economic aftermath of divorce (Lesthaeghe, 2003). Most importantly, women have moved into the workforce en masse: 68% of women with children under the age of 18 were in the civilian labor force in 2008 (Bureau of Labor Statistics, 2009). Women are the primary caregivers for family members with disabilities, a fact that has changed little since the 19th century, despite major changes in employment, marriage patterns, and child rearing. In 2009, 60% of all care recipients were related to their caregivers as parents, siblings, spouses or children; 69% of all care recipients had a long-term disability (NAC, 2009). Almost 70% of all caregivers were women and only 69% of these female caregivers were employed compared to 82% of male caregivers. Cultural values and the momentum of history account for this dual role. For many women, the labor of caregiving is performed for their own children and their elderly parents at the same time because of increased longevity and delayed childbearing. In a recent study of women in the "sandwich generation," those caring for two generations of family members, many also reported caring for their in-laws, too (Hammer & Neal, 2008). At the same time that the population is aging, families are smaller, more women are single parents, and more are impoverished as a result of divorce. This scenario of increased demand in an era of decreased capacity threatens to reduce the quality of life for many women. Feminist scholars have expressed the concern that the intensification of caregiving demands may recapitulate traditional domestic roles and further reify oppression of women (Aronson & Neysmith, 1997). One important rationale for creating new supports for caregiving families is based on concern for equity, so that taken-for-granted traditional roles do not further diminish the quality of life for women in caregiving families.

The value placed on residing at home and receiving care from loved ones reflects the social construction of the home in the United States and Europe, one that developed as recently as the mid-19th century (Hareven, 1977). The preference for home as a place to give and receive care is deeply embedded in U.S. majority culture. It is a taken-for-granted assumption made by policy makers, advocates, and caregivers that most elderly individuals and people with disabilities greatly prefer to remain in their own homes rather than reside in nursing homes or other congregate care arrangements. Since the 1970s, individuals with disabilities have organized to advocate for public funding for personal assistance services and consumer-controlled financial assistance specifically to help with the costs of living at home in the community (Powers, Sowers, & Singer, 2006).

Although women's roles in the United States have changed profoundly in the economic and educational realms, there has been less change in the allocation of caregiving and homemaking labor. The division of labor and locus of the separate spheres was bolstered by an ideology that placed nurture, care, self-expression, and intimacy within the boundaries of the private home whereas struggle, competition, and the impersonal characteristics of the technical/rationale structuring of the factory and the corporation were enacted by men at the workplace (Kerber, 1988). The social construction of the idealized home frames it as a place of refuge, for private fulfillment, a realm of affection, a sense of belonging, and the place for the exercise of self-determination and individualism. Women were expected to manage and do most of the work in the home side of the separate realms. Women's work in the home included the primary responsibility for raising children and caring for an ill or relative with disabilities. However, this work, although essential to any society, was devalued (Orloff, 2002). The ideal of the home as a place of refuge, and personalization is taken for granted in much of the policy discourse about caregiving, as is the unstated assumption that women will do the caregiving work (Aronson & Neysmith, 1997).

One reason for the taken-for-granted transfer of caregiving work to women has to do with the nature of caregiving itself. By definition individuals with the most severe disabilities are those people who require extensive assistance with basic life activities, activities of daily living. These are the very activities that have traditionally fallen under the purview of women in their role as mothers of young children. Such tasks as meal preparation, feeding, shopping for clothing and food, grooming, dressing, and bathing were traditionally managed by mothers. When adults with disabilities need assistance with these same tasks they are assumed to also be the job of women.

In the value system underlying the separate spheres, whenever possible, care for ill, elderly, and individuals with disabilities was to be performed and received in the home where norms of intimacy, presence, and individualization were to prevail for care recipients, usually under the care of their female relatives (Baker, 2008). Caregiving not only encompassed the many tasks of helping family members with disabilities with daily activities but also involved emotion work (Rae, 1998). When families could not provide care, a residual population of people with disabilities was transferred to asylums, hospitals, and nursing homes where they were attended by low-wage workers. The vast majority of informal caregiving since the 19th century has been gendered, unpaid, and home based. An estimate of the contemporary economic value of unpaid home caregiving in the United States was an estimated $375 billion in 2007 (Houser & Gibson, 2008).

The economic, social, and family situations of women have changed profoundly since the gendered division of labor around caregiving was first established as a norm. Although women's roles outside of the home have changed profoundly, change has been much slower within the household. Although women made up almost one half of the U.S. workforce in Fall 2009, they continue to perform most household work including caregiving for relatives with disabilities (NAC, 2009). Household work has been characterized as "the second shift" for employed women, who performed an average of 26.7 hours of unpaid work per week in the years 2003 to 2007 (Krantz-Kent, 2009). When women also devote substantial amounts of time to caregiving for relatives with disabilities, the workload increases, along with the risk of stress-related physical and psychological problems. Currently, in the United States roughly 66% of caregivers and 62% of care recipients are female (NAC, 2009). Men have gradually been taking up a significant portion of caregiving with fewer hours and often less emotionally demanding duties than women assume. When men give care to relatives with disabilities, they perform work that is often less intimate and, arguably, requires less emotion work. Compared to the care that women provide, men are much less likely to help a relative with disabilities to dress, bathe, groom, or prepare a meal (Kramer & Kipnis, 1995).

In summary, the expectation that women care for relatives with disabilities in family homes was established under very different economic and social conditions than prevail at present. Social norms about the importance of home living and the centrality of women as caregivers have changed little despite radical changes in their social and economic circumstances. At the same time the numbers and proportion of people with disabilities in the United States is growing dramatically. Under these conditions the impetus for new social arrangements to support family caregiving can only grow.

ECONOMIC TRENDS

Given the demands of paid employment outside the home and unpaid labor within it, U.S. citizens with sufficient income have transferred traditional household work to the private economy (Coltrane, 2000). Increasingly meals are prepared and eaten outside of the home rather than in family kitchens, and families with young children pay for childcare, making employment possible (Kant & Graubard, 2004). When they can afford it, many caregiving families elect to purchase caregiving services for their relatives. Social class is a key factor in the extent to which family caregivers are able to transfer some of the work of caregiving to paid help; 30% of caregiving households with incomes below $50,000 a year use some paid help compared to 48% with incomes above $100,000 (NAC, 2009).

The paid nursing home and home care workforce is one of the most important determinants in the quality of life of people with disabilities (Stone & Wiener, 2001). In the United States most paid caregiving jobs are performed by paraprofessionals who are low-wage workers with relatively low levels of education (Kuttner, 2008). Turnover rates in home care workers are high; most are not represented by unions and have little power to bargain with their employers, although when states have passed legislation promoting union organizing of home care workers, pay levels have improved substantially (Kuttner, 2008; Stone & Wiener, 2001). These jobs are often held by immigrant women, some of whom are undocumented workers that are even more vulnerable to deliberate or inadvertent exploitation. The latter may arise when caregiving tasks are unfinished at the end of a paid caregiving session and informal bonds of obligation compel home care workers to continue working unpaid (Aronson & Neysmith, 1996).

When caregivers are caught between demands at work and caregiving, they are at risk of becoming less productive. Asked about the impact of caregiving on their outside employment, a large majority of caregivers in the NAC (2009) survey reported that they had to go to work late, leave early, or take unpaid time off to deal with caregiving demands. In 2006, the estimated cost to businesses for family caregiving employees was more than $33 billion annually (MMI, 2010; MMI & NAC, 2006). Employers and consumers accrue these costs in the context of a period of rapid inflation in the costs of health insurance. At times of economic downturn employers and employees are likely to be more stressed by the demands of employees' dual roles. For the millions of individuals who become unemployed, the extra fiscal costs that have been documented in caregiving become all the more challenging. These and other macroeconomic trends also highlight the importance of informal caregiving in the long-term care system.

It is widely agreed that, absent extensive reform, the costs of Medicaid, Medicare, and Social Security, the primary federal programs providing resources for supporting family caregivers, will become unsupportable by midcentury (Social Security Administration, 2009). As U.S. political parties and interest groups address looming costs, one likely strategy for cost saving will be to boost the capacity of informal caregivers to support elderly citizens. The value placed on cost savings cuts two ways; on one hand, political pressure to reduce public expenditures has fueled efforts to support family caregiving as a less costly alternative to institutional placement. On the other hand, this rationale greatly limits the numbers of families eligible for assistance with caregiving. It perforce places the goal of cost reduction as more important than other social benefits of providing high quality family support. Furthermore, if federal funding for bolstering home care depends on a rhetorical commitment to cost reduction of long-term care, the costs cannot be justified if evidence indicates such savings are not in fact realized.

States are also experimenting with a relatively new approach to designing services that, in some cases, address the needs of caregivers and care receivers. Medicaid Cash and Counseling programs have tested the option of giving family caregivers and people with disabilities the same amount of autonomy and control over resources as do people with private funds (Doty, 1998). As a corollary of the movement for personal care assistance, advocates have lobbied for changes in rules that govern who can receive and administer public payments. Small-scale consumer directed programs under Medicaid waiver programs have allowed consumers to hire their own assistants. Traditional service design gives control of funds to top–down agencies rather than to consumers. This approach grows out of faith in top-down approaches originally designed to maintain social control and is rooted in distrust of aid recipients as decision makers, an attitude that has been a longstanding premise in the political culture in the United States. It is eroding under pressure of social changes directly associated with the disability rights movement and indirectly from the transformation of the roles of women as caregivers as a result of changes in women's social roles.

A striking feature of these social experiments is that in some cases they allow public funds to be used to pay family members to provide care. For example, California's In-Home Supportive Services Program (IHSS) provides funds directly to individuals with eligible disabilities or over 65 who may elect to pay family members for caregiving. Evaluations of these pilot programs have been positive for people with disabilities and their informal caregivers (Sciegaj, Simone, & Mahoney, 2007). When offered a choice between agency-directed and self-directed services, caregivers and people with disabilities frequently choose the latter option. In an evaluation of self-directed programs in three states, a randomized trial was used to test the impact of the model compared to the traditional top-down approach (Doty, 1998). The results were very positive in terms of physical and psychological outcomes for the consumers with disabilities as well as for their informal caregivers. Informal caregivers reported significantly less stress, less worry about the care recipient, increased well-being, and better health. The evaluation study also found this model was more expensive than the traditional one during the first few years of operation, but that costs differences leveled out over time, making the programs at least cost-neutral (Feinberg, Wolkwitz, & Goldstein, 2006). In a few states, family members can be paid for providing services that otherwise would have to be purchased (Feinberg & Newman, 2004). Similar experiments are underway in at least 22 states in Medicare programs which are testing wrap-around capitated care models of support. The Program of All-Inclusive Care for the Elderly (PACE) allows interdisciplinary teams to allocate funds to provide respite care, counseling, and additional hours for community center attendance to alleviate family caregivers' stress. A fixed budget combining federal, state, and private funds is formulated to create individualized mixes of services and supports for keeping elderly people who are at risk for nursing home placement in their own homes. These models recognize as a matter of policy and public commitment of resources that family caregivers are an essential element of comprehensive programs for the elderly.

Medicaid and Medicare continues to have an institutional bias, with greater amounts allocated for nursing homes for the elderly than for home care despite an overwhelming difference in the numbers of elderly individuals supported by relatives compared to those who live in institutions. In 1999, Medicaid spent $72 billion on institutional care compared to just over $16 billion for home and community-based care (Doty, 2000). The great preponderance of Medicare funds for residential costs of elderly citizens go to nursing home and are administered by agencies rather than care recipients or their families.

INCREMENTALISM, FRAGMENTATION, AND THE EVOLUTION OF THE WELFARE STATE

Public policy regarding governmental support for family caregiving has been characterized by piecemeal programs of relatively small scope marked by a lack of consistency and coordination. This fragmentation is partly due to the political processes that have created family support programs and partly because of the way diagnostic categorization has predominated in the ways caregiving has been conceptualized and how special interest groups have organized to lobby for public resources. Until the most recent decade, most of this political advocacy, and the polices resulting from it, have been organized based on the category of disability affecting the family member who requires care. Similarly, the scholarly disciplines studying family caregiving have usually been organized around diagnostic categories or age levels of individuals with disabilities although there have been some notable efforts at cross-cutting categorical analysis (Biegel & Schulz, 1991–1996). For the most part, scholarship and services have developed separately despite the fact that many of the needs families have for help with caregiving are shared in common, regardless of why a family member requires extra levels of assistance in daily life.

Recent initiatives include the use of assessments of caregivers in the planning of individual services. New assessment systems have been developed for determining the needs of families as well as the primary recipients of support (Feinberg et al., 2006). This trend is important because it is another step in recognizing the family as a key part a network of support for a community-based system of long-term care.

CONVERGENCE IN SUPPORT PROGRAMS AND PUBLIC POLICY

Policy fragmentation and incrementalism have begun to give way to more universal and larger scope policy efforts led by coalitions with shared interests in family support. A notable result of coalition efforts is the Lifespan Respite Care Act of 2006. It amended the Public Health Service Act to create a national funding stream for States to establish coordinated systems of respite care for families of children and adults with disabilities. The life-span approach stands in marked contrast to the previous history of age-specific policies. The Act provides for information and referral services, support for respite care provision, and training for family members in caregiving. In response to a NAC (2009) national survey, family caregivers listed respite care as one of their most preferred forms of government assistance, regardless of the age or disability of the care recipient. Because of a shared interest in the development of a national respite policy, the Access to Respite Care and Help (ARCH) National Respite Coalition working group, Lifespan Respite Task Force, was formed. In 2006, the Lifespan Respite Task Force was comprised of over 150 national, state and local organizations advocating for caregivers of people with a multitude of different conditions who were a driving force behind the Lifespan Respite Act of 2006 (ARCH National Respite Coalition, 2006, 2009). Coalition members, for example, included the Alzheimer's Association and the Children's Defence Fund (ARCH, 2006). The Lifespan Respite Act of 2006 signals the advent of national legislative and policy recognition that a substantial portion of what families need is likely to be shared regardless of the cause of a family member's disability.

In large part, this commonality exists because the functional activities and routines that occur in most family homes are similar, as are the particular support provisions that benefit caregivers (Singer & Powers, 1993). When asked about what programs and policies they would most like to see enacted, respondents to the NAC (2009) endorsed, in order of preference: (1) a policy that would provide a $3,000 tax credit for caregivers, (2) a voucher that would pay family members minimum wage for at least some of the hours spent on caregiving, (3) respite services that would allow caregivers to take a break, and (4) an outside service to provide transportation for care recipients. All of these preferences would likely be of benefit regardless of the disability category and most efficiently addressed with a broad national mandate.

The Lifespan Respite Care Act of 2006 appealed to legislators on the Left inclined to expand government services in response to changes in population demographics, employment, and social values regarding the roles of women in the public and private spheres. At the same time, it appealed to those on the Right who wanted to restrict government by paying for the lesser expense of respite care, instead of the much greater cost of institutionalization. This unusual coalition of Left and Right was united by appeal to at least two values: (1) the belief that home care is preferable to institutional care, a widely held value in U.S. culture, and (2) the belief in the need to conserve or limit public spending. Congress members endorsing the Act argued that there would be large cost savings. Advocates for the Act argued that costly out-of-home placement for people with disabilities can be delayed or prevented by providing respite for caregivers. For example, in a study of events precipitating nursing home placements, Gaugler, Leach, Clay, and Newcomer (2004) found that elderly people were much less likely to move into nursing homes if primary caregivers, usually spouses, had other family members who provided overnight relief from caregiving and helped with activities of daily living such as shopping for groceries and transportation to appointments. The national respite care legislation aimed to address some of these needs through purchased services.

At this time, both houses of Congress have passed legislation with long-term care provisions expressly aimed at allowing individuals with disabilities to remain in their own homes and control their own care. If this new program, the result of decades of advocacy, comes to fruition, the use of a national insurance program to meet the growing needs of individuals with disabilities and their caregivers will shift historically and make a major difference in the lives of millions of people. The impact that policy or its absence can have on whole populations of citizens can be seen in the current condition of services for individuals with developmental disabilities compared to a group of people who often have similar needs for supports, individuals with serious mental illnesses.

THE DIFFERENCE SOCIAL POLICY CAN MAKE FOR CAREGIVERS AND PEOPLE WHO RECEIVE CARE

There are alternatives to the residualist model. A more fine-grained analysis of the use of Medicaid home and community based services (HCBS) waiver funds across different populations and different states reveals the impact of alternative values and political will as the basis for design of public assistance for family caregiving. Since the late 1960s, advocates for individuals with developmental disabilities have fought for deinstitutionalization and creation of an array of community living options. Medicaid has a powerful institutional bias, even with the availability of waivers; almost one half of the Medicaid budget is spent on the less than 4% of the population residing in state hospitals. Nonetheless, consistent advocacy and political support for community alternatives have created real alternatives for many people with mental retardation. The idea greatly influencing these efforts was the principle of normalization. Wolfensberger (1972) argued that the state should provide assistance for people with intellectual disabilities in culturally normative settings using culturally normative means. Hence, the places where they should live, work, and play ought to be in the community. Accordingly, children should live in their families' homes rather than institutions, and adults should live in small home-like residences with necessary supports to live a high quality of life including meaningful employment and recreational opportunities. Most states made use of matching state and federal Medicaid HCBS waivers to create at least basic systems of community services and supports. These have included funds for supporting families of children with severe disabilities living at home.

Rather than a residualist ethic, the driving rationale has been the recognition of the basic civil rights of people with cognitive disabilities, including the right to normal life in the community rather than segregation and seclusion in institutions. In the Americans with Disabilities Act of 1990, Congress found that "individuals with disabilities are a discrete and insular minority who have been faced with restrictions and limitations, subjected to a history of purposeful unequal treatment, and relegated to a position of political powerlessness in our society" (42 U.S.C. §12101(a)(7)). The ADA Amendments Act of 2008 amended this and other findings, including the finding that "physical or mental disabilities in no way diminish a person's right to fully participate in all aspects of society" (42 U.S.C. §12101(a)(1)). The U.S. Supreme Court lent additional authority to this movement, ruling in *Olmstead v L.C.* (1999) that people with developmental disabilities living in institutional settings had a right to life in the community if an interdisciplinary team determines that community living is appropriate. This decision prompted many states to develop plans for moving the remainder of their institutionalized populations out into the community, accelerating a long-standing trend.

Beginning in the early 1990s, combined federal and state expenditures for community living options for people with developmental disabilities exceeded spending on large institutions, a policy known as "rebalancing," an effort to change the balance of funding from a preponderance of spending on institutions to a more equitable allocation for community services (Lakin & Prouty, 2003). However, as of 2000, only 4% of funds for people with developmental disabilities were allocated for family support to help sustain family caregiving. Four percent represents growth from the 1.5% allocated in 1990 (Parish, Pomeranz-Essley, & Braddock, 2003), but it is miniscule compared to the substantial extra costs of home caregiving for family members with developmental disabilities. Family caregiving has only recently been considered an essential part of the community system of care that is worthy of public funding. The health care reforms of 2010 do recognize this need with the creation of a new long term care insurance fund, which allows for payments to family members for certain forms of caregiving. By basing the development of a system on Medicaid waivers and matching state funds, the service system has necessarily emphasized services for people who could plausibly be described as most likely to be institutionalized. Although advocates and their allies have been creative in using this approach to ensure many services are available to people with developmental disabilities, residualist policy restrictions have limited full development, leaving immense unmet needs (Rizzolo, Hemp, Braddock, & Schindler, 2009).

In response to effective advocacy from family organizations, states began to establish community alternatives for individuals with developmental disabilities in the mid-1960s. A few states have provided cash stipends for family caregivers since the 1980s, and most have regional service centers providing case management, person centered planning, respite care, evaluation services, and access to a variety of supported living and employment options.

By contrast, most states have done much less for individuals with serious mental illness and their families. Medicaid waivers were rarely used to fund services for persons with mental illness, partly because different sources of funding, including the Community Mental Health Centers Act of 1963, were supposed to help states establish community alternatives to mental hospitals. However, this endeavor was never sufficiently funded; at the same time, public mental hospitals were closed down, usually to save costs but with lip service given to promoting community living. There was not a concomitant effort to create a community system, as was done for persons with developmental disabilities. Families have in large part been left to fend for themselves in caring for family members with serious mental illness, as very few community options were available in large sections of the United States (Aron et al., 2009). Rubin (2007) describes the experiences of many families:

> Ask any family with a schizophrenic or bipolar member, and you'll hear stories about the weird and sometimes dangerous behavior that suddenly appears when the patient secretly stops taking medication. Listen to them speak of the difficulty of finding their way through the chaotic maze of uncoordinated public agencies that is now our mental health system, only to fail because there are no beds or community services available. Hear their agony as they describe what it's like to find a loved one living on the street and be helpless to do anything about it. (p. 54–55)

Tragically, the facilities that hold the largest groups of people with serious mental illness in the United States are state prisons and county jails such as in Los Angeles and New York City (Teplin, 1990). The divergent impact of contrary social policies can also be seen in the effects of family caregivers. A 30-year longitudinal comparison of families of individuals with intellectual disabilities and families of individuals with serious mental illnesses found that the former group of families were significantly better off by the end of the study (Seltzer, Greenberg, Floyd, Pettee, & Hong, 2001). Parents of adult children with mental illness were in poorer physical health and had higher levels of depressive symptoms and rates of problems with alcohol. It is important to note, however, that some of the costs of family caregiving for people with intellectual disabilities were also revealed. Caregivers of adults with intellectual disabilities had lower occupational achievement, less employment, and less social participation than a control group of parents of adults without disabilities, though psychological well-being, rates of divorce, and educational attainment were normative.

IS CHANGE ON ITS WAY?

Currently, both houses of Congress have passed health care reform bills containing a proposed mandate that was originally an independent bill, the Community Living Assistance Services and Supports Act (CLASS Act) (S. 697

and H.R. 1721). It would create a new national long-term care insurance program paid for voluntarily through payroll taxes. Funds from this insurance would be used to help people with functional limitations live in their own homes, remain as independent as possible, and have control of how their public insurance funds are used. The bills from both sides of Congress expressly allow funds to be given to family members to pay them for some of the costs of caring for a relative with physical or mental disabilities, regardless of the age of the family members and the causes of the disabilities. Unlike most previous legislation, it is a noncategorical program. Whether the CLASS Act becomes law in 2010, initiatives similar to it will likely either remain visible or resurface in the future because the trends and forces that have placed it on the public agenda are persistent and will inevitably increase.

In summary, social and economic trends are bringing the issue of support for family caregiving to the public agenda. At the same time that there is an increase in the absolute numbers and relative proportion of people of all ages with disabilities living in the community, families' human and fiscal resources for caregiving have eroded, resulting in considerable stress and distress. The residualist tradition in the U.S. welfare state has led to an emphasis on nursing homes and other congregate care facilities over support for community living. This bias is being challenged by advocates for people with disabilities and their informal caregivers. The cultural value placed on the home and on personal autonomy in the majority culture in the United States has collided with the top-down approach of agency control of decision making about the use of public funds and a bias toward institutional living. Despite a tradition of piecemeal development of services for people from categorical disability groups, there is a growing convergence in policy goals and in the intervention research literature. These forces are likely to remain at play and increase over the next decade as the number of elderly people and individuals with long-term chronic conditions in the United States increases.

REFERENCES

Access to Respite Care and Help, National Respite Coalition. (2006). *National, state and local organizations endorsing the "Lifespan Respite Care Act of 2005"*. Retrieved March 11, 2010, from http://www.archrespite.org/JointEndorsingList.pdf

Access to Respite Care and Help, National Respite Coalition. (2009). *National Respite Coalition Lifespan Respite Task Force*. Retrieved March 11, 2010, from http://chtop.org/ARCH/Lifespan-Respite-Task-Force.html

ADA Amendments Act of 2008, 42 U.S.C. §12101 *et seq.*

Americans with Disabilities Act of 1990, 42 U.S.C. §12101 *et seq.*

Aron, L., Honberg, R., Duckworth, K., Kimball, A., Edgar, E., Carolla, B., et al. (2009). *Grading the states 2009: A report on America's health care system for adults with serious mental illness*. Retrieved March 10, 2010, from the National Alliance on Mental Illness Web site: http://www.nami.org/gtsTemplate09.cfm?Section=Grading_the_States_2009&Template=/ContentManagement/ContentDisplay.cfm&ContentID=75459

Aronson, J., & Neysmith, S. M. (1997). The retreat of the state and long-term care provision: Implications for frail elderly people, unpaid family carers and paid home care workers. *Studies in Political Economy, 53*, 37–66.

Baker, J. (2008). All things considered, should feminists embrace basic income? *Basic Income Studies, 3*(3), Article 6. Retrieved March 11, 2010, from http://www.bepress.com/bis/vol3/iss3/art6

Biegel, D. E., Sales, E., & Schulz, R. (1991). *Family caregiving in chronic illness: Alzheimer's disease, cancer, heart disease, mental illness and stroke*. Newbury Park, CA: Sage.

Biegel, D. E. & Schulz, R. (Series Eds.). (1991–1996). *Family caregiver applications* (Vols. 1–7). Newbury Park, CA: Sage.

Bureau of Labor Statistics. (2009). *Women in the labor force: A Databook* (Report 1018). Retrieved March 10, 2010, from http://www.bls.gov/cps/wlf-databook-2009.pdf

Coltrane, S. (2000). Research on household labor: Modeling and measuring the social embeddedness of routine family work. *Journal of Marriage and the Family, 62*(4), 1208–1233.

Community Living Assistance Services and Supports Act of 2009. H.R. 1721, 111th Cong. (2009).

Community Living Assistance Services and Supports Act of 2009. S. 697. 111th Cong. (2009).

Doty, P. (2000). *Cost-effectiveness of home and community-based long-term care services*. Retrieved March 10, 2010, from US Department of Health and Human Services Web site: http://aspe.hhs.gov/daltcp/reports/costeff.htm

Doty, P. J. (1998). The Cash and Counseling Demonstration: An experiment in consumer-directed personal assistance services. *American Rehabilitation, 24*(3), 27–30.

Feinberg, L. F., & Newman, S. L. (2004). A study of 10 states since passage of the National Family Caregiver Support Program: Policies, perceptions, and program development. *Gerontologist, 44*(6), 760–769.

Feinberg, L. F., Wolkwitz, K., & Goldstein, C. (2006). *Ahead of the curve: Emerging trends and practices in family caregiver support* (AARP Public Policy Institute Issue Paper #2006–09). Washington, DC: AARP. Retrieved March 11, 2010, from http://assets.aarp.org/rgcenter/il/inb120_caregiver.pdf

Gaugler, J. E., Leach, C. R., Clay, T., & Newcomer, R. C. (2004). Predictors of nursing home placement in African Americans with dementia. *Journal of the American Geriatrics Society, 52*(3), 445–452.

Hammer, L. B., & Neal, M. B. (2008). Working sandwiched-generation caregivers: Prevalence, characteristics, and outcomes. *The Psychologist-Manager, 11*(1), 93–112.

Hareven, T. K. (1977). Family time and historical time. *Deadelus, 106*(2), 57–70.

Hastings, R. P., & Taunt, H. M. (2002). Positive perceptions in families of children with developmental disabilities. *American Journal on Mental Retardation, 107*(2), 116–127.

Houser, A., & Gibson, M. J. (2008). Valuing the invaluable: The economic value of family caregiving, 2008 update. *AARP Public Policy Institute: Insight on the Issues, 13*. Retrieved March 11, 2010, from http://assets.aarp.org/rgcenter/il/i13_caregiving.pdf

Hughes, S. L., Gobbie-Hurder, A., Weaver, F. M., & Hendersen, W. (1999). Relationship between caregiver burden and health-related quality of life. *Gerontologist, 39*(5), 534–545.

Kant, A. K., & Graubard, B. I. (2004). Eating out in America, 1987–2000: Trends and nutritional correlates. *Preventive Medicine, 38*(2), 243–249.

Kerber, L. K. (1988). Separate spheres, female worlds, woman's place: The rhetoric of women's history. *Journal of American History, 75*(1), 9–39.

Kramer, B. J., & Kipnis, S. (1995). Eldercare and work-role conflict: Toward an understanding of gender differences in caregiver burden. *Gerontologist, 35*(3), 340–348.

Krantz-Kent, R. (2009). Measuring time spent in unpaid household work: Results from the American Time Use Survey. *Monthly Labor Review, 132*(7), 46–59.

Kuttner, R. (2008). *Obama's challenge: America's economic crisis and the power of a transformative presidency*. White River Junction, VT: Chelsea Green Publishing.

Lakin, K. C., & Prouty, R. (2003). *Medicaid home and community-based services: The first 20 years*. (Policy Research Brief, 14(3)). Minneapolis, MN: University of Minnesota, Institute on Community Integration. Retrieved March 10, 2010, from University of Minnesota, Institute on Community Integration Web site: http://ici.umn.edu/products/prb/143/143.pdf

Lesthaeghe, R. (2003). The second demographic transition in Western countries: An interpretation. In K. O. Mason & A.-M. Jensen (Eds.), *Gender and family change in industrialized countries* (pp. 17–62). New York: Oxford University Press.

Lifespan Respite Care Act of 2006, 101, Pub. L. No. 109-442. 1, 42 USC 201 (2006).

MetLife Mature Market Institute. (2006). *The MetLife study of Alzheimer's disease: The caregiving experience*. Westport, CT: MetLife Mature Market Institute. Retrieved March 1, 2010, from http://www.metlife.com/assets/cao/mmi/publications/studies/mmi-alzheimers-disease-caregiving-experience-study.pdf

MetLife Mature Market Institute. (2010). *The MetLife study of working caregivers and employer health care costs*. Westport, CT: MetLife Mature Market Institute. Retrieved March 1, 2010, from http://www.metlife.com/assets/cao/mmi/publications/studies/2010/mmi-working-caregivers-employers-health-care-costs.pdf

MetLife Mature Market Institute, & National Alliance for Caregiving. (2006). *The MetLife caregiving cost study: Productivity losses to U.S. business*. Westport, CT: MetLife Mature Market Institute. Retrieved from National Alliance for Caregiving Web site April 27, 2010, from http://www.caregiving.org/data/Caregiver%20Cost%20Study.pdf

National Alliance for Caregiving. (2009). *Caregiving in the U.S. 2009*. Retrieved February 2, 2010, from http://assets.aarp.org/rgcenter/il/caregiving_09_fr.pdf

Olmstead v. L. C., 527 U.S. 581 (1999).

Orloff, A. S. (2002). Explaining US welfare reform: Power, gender, race and the US policy legacy. *Critical Social Policy, 22*(1), 96–118.

Parish, S. L., Pomeranz-Essley, A., & Braddock, D. (2003). Family support in the United States: Financing trends and emerging initiatives. *Mental Retardation, 41*(3), 174–187.

Pinquart, M., & Sörensen, S. (2004). Associations of caregiver stressors and uplifts with subjective well-being and depressive mood: A meta-analytic comparison. *Aging and Mental Health, 8*(5), 438–449.

Powers, L. E., Sowers, J.-A., & Singer, G. H. S. (2006). A cross-disability analysis of person-directed, long-term services. *Journal of Disability Policy Studies, 17*(2), 66–76.

Rae, H. M. (1998). Managing feelings caregiving as emotion work. *Research on Aging, 20*(1), 137–160.

Rizzolo, M. C., Hemp, R., Braddock, D., & Schindler, A. (2009). Family support services for persons with intellectual and developmental disabilities: Recent national trends. *Intellectual and Developmental Disabilities, 47*(2), 152–155.

Rubin, L. B. (2007). Sand castles and snake pits: Homelessness, public policy, and the law of unintended consequences. *Dissent, 54*(5), 51–56.

Sciegaj, M., Simone, K., & Mahoney, K. (2007). State experiences with implementing the Cash and Counseling Demonstration and Evaluation project. *Journal of Aging & Social Policy, 20*(1), 81–98.

Schulze, B., & Rössler, W. (2005). Caregiver burden in mental illness: Review of measurement, findings and interventions in 2004–2005. *Current Opinion in Psychiatry, 18*(6), 684–691.

Seltzer, M. A., Greenberg, J. S., Floyd, F. J., Pettee, Y., & Hong, J. (2001). Life course impacts of parenting a child with a disability. *American Journal on Mental Retardation, 106*(3), 265–286.

Singer, G. H. S. (2006). Meta-analysis of comparative studies of depression in mothers of children with and without developmental disabilities. *American Journal on Mental Retardation, 111*(3), 155–169.

Singer, G. H. S., & Powers, L. E. (1993). Contributing to resilience in families: An overview. In G. H. S. Singer & L. E. Powers (Eds.), *Families, disability, and empowerment: Active coping skills and strategies for family interventions* (pp. 1–26). Baltimore, MD: Paul H. Brookes Publishing.

Social Security Administration. (2009). *A summary of the 2009 Annual Reports: Social Security and Medicare Boards of Trustees*. Retrieved March 9, 2010, from http://www.socialsecurity.gov/OACT/TRSUM/

Social Security Administration. (2010). *Reference Supplemental Security Income (SSI) in California* (SSA Publication No. 05-11125). Retrieved March 10, 2010, from http://ftp.ssa.gov/pubs/11125.pdf

Stone, R. I., & Wiener, J. M. (2001). *Who will care for us? Addressing the long-term care workforce crisis*. Washington, DC: Urban Institute and American Association of Homes and Services for the Aging. Retrieved March 9, 2010, from http://www.urban.org/UploadedPDF/Who_will_Care_for_Us.pdf

Teplin, L. A. (1990). The prevalence of severe mental disorder among male urban jail detainees: Comparison with the Epidemiologic Catchment Area program. *American Journal of Public Health, 80*(6), 663–669.

Wolfensberger, W. (1972). *The principle of normalization in human services*. Toronto, Canada: National Institute on Mental Retardation.

Index

Page numbers in *Italics* represent tables.
Page numbers in **Bold** represent figures.